Practical Pulmonary Rehabilitation

D0626158

Practical Pulmonary Rehabilitation

Edited by

Mike Morgan

Consultant Physician
Department of Respiratory Medicine and Thoracic Surgery
Glenfield Hospital
Leicester, UK

and

Sally Singh

Pulmonary Rehabilitation Co-ordinator
Department of Respiratory Medicine and Thoracic Surgery
Glenfield Hospital
Leicester, UK

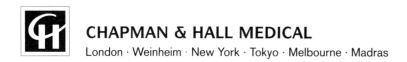

CHAPMAN & HALL MEDICAL

London · Weinheim · New York · Tokyo · Melbourne · Madras

Published by Chapman & Hall, 2-6 Boundary Row, London SE1 8HN, UK

Chapman & Hall, 2-6 Boundary Row, London SE1 8HN, UK

Chapman & Hall GmbH, Pappelallee 3, 69469 Weinheim, Germany

Chapman & Hall USA, 115 Fifth Avenue, New York, NY 10003, USA

Chapman & Hall Japan, ITP-Japan, Kyowa Building, 3F, 2-2-1 Hirakawacho, Chiyoda-ku, Tokyo 102, Japan

Chapman & Hall Australia, 102 Dodds Street, South Melbourne, Victoria 3205, Australia

Chapman & Hall India, R. Seshadri, 32 Second Main Road, CIT East, Madras 600 035, India

First edition 1997

© 1997 Chapman & Hall

Typeset in 10/13 pt Meridien by Best-set Typesetter Ltd., Hong Kong

ISBN 0 412 61810 9

In memory of Trevor Clay who lived with lung disease

Contents

List of contributors   ix

Foreword   xi

1. Practical pulmonary rehabilitation: an introduction   1
   MDL Morgan

2. Patient selection and assessment for pulmonary
   rehabilitation   19
   SJ Singh

3. Assessment of quality of life in chronic lung disease   49
   ME Hyland

4. Exercise training   63
   (a) Theoretical rationale for training   65
   AE Hardman
   (b) Aerobic exercise training in patients with COPD   81
   SJ Singh
   (c) Inspiratory muscle training   99
   RS Goldstein
   (d) Isolated muscle training in respiratory rehabilitation   117
   DG Stubbing

5. Nutrition – theoretical background and practical advice   127
   J Congleton
   Appendix 5A. Treating poor appetite and weight loss   151
   S Pitten and S Patel

6. Physiotherapy   155
   J Bott

7. Lifestyle management: relaxation, coping, sex, benefits and travel   179
   S Gibson

8. Disease education and medical support   213
   MDL Morgan

9. The role of the respiratory nurse and home care   237
    A Heslop

10. Palliation of non-malignant disease   255
    S Ahmedzai

Appendix A: Abbreviations   273
Appendix B: Useful Addresses   275
Index   277

Contributors

Prof S Ahmedzai
Palliative Medicine Section
The University of Sheffield
K Floor
Royal Hallamshire Hospital
Sheffield S10 2JF

Ms J Bott
Head of Research and Development
Physiotherapy Department
Royal Brompton Hospital
Sydney Street
London SW3 6NP

Dr J Congleton
Chelsea and Westminster Hospital
369 Fulham Road
London SW10 9NH

Ms S Gibson
Occupational Therapy Advisor (South
    District)
Hinckley Sunny-Side Hospital
Ashby Road
Hinckley
Leicestershire LE10 3AD

Dr RS Goldstein
Professor of Medicine
University of Toronto
c/o West Park Hospital
82 Buttonwood Avenue
Toronto
Ontario M6M 2JS
Canada

Dr AE Hardman
Reader in Human Exercise Metabolism
Department of Physical Education, Sports
    Science and Recreation Management
Loughborough University
Loughborough
Leicestershire LE11 3TU

Ms A Heslop
c/o PO Box 791
Hermanus 7200
Cape
South Africa

Prof ME Hyland
Department of Psychology
University of Plymouth
Drake Circus
Plymouth
Devon PL4 8AA

Dr MDL Morgan
Consultant Physician
Department of Respiratory Medicine and
    Thoracic Surgery
The Glenfield Hospital
Groby Road
Leicester LE3 9QP

Dr SJ Singh
Pulmonary Rehabilitation Co-ordinator
Department of Respiratory Medicine and
    Thoracic Surgery
The Glenfield Hospital
Groby Road
Leicester LE3 9QP

Dr DG Stubbing
Associate Professor
Department of Medicine
McMaster University and
    Hamilton Health Science Corporation
Hamilton
Ontario
Canada

Foreword

In the past, the emphasis of management of patients with chronic lung disease has been on the prevention of deterioration and the reversal of impairment by drug therapy. Scant attention has been paid to the needs of patients to live with their disability. This climate is now beginning to change with the realization that something useful can be done to improve the quality of life in those who sufferer from such a common condition. In addition, there has been the development of appropriate methods of assessment in the areas of functional performance and quality of life. These more subtle measurements have allowed researchers to identify and quantify benefits which had previously only been subjective. The art of rehabilitation in chronic lung disease has given way to scientific understanding, exploration and development.

We hope that this book is a timely review of the progress that has been made in the field of pulmonary rehabilitation. We have not set out to reiterate the details of conventional management of lung disease. To that end the reader may feel that there are omissions in the descriptions of topical subjects such as oxygen therapy, non-invasive ventilation or lung volume reduction surgery. Our intention is to concentrate on those aspects of care which improve physical and social functioning beyond that which could be regarded as normal clinic or hospital care. The aim is to provide the reader with a theoretical background complemented by practical advice on how to develop a rehabilitation programme. The work is multi-disciplinary in scope and should present an opportunity to all health care professionals to experience the working practices and language of their colleagues.

Rehabilitation has much to offer the individual patient and the professions that deal with lung disease. We fully acknowledge that much scientific work is required to understand the mechanisms and potential benefits of pulmonary rehabilitation. However the evidence of benefit can only be obtained if investment and funding follow enthusiasm. We hope that this book can encourage others to begin that process.

MDL Morgan & SJ Singh May 1997

1. Practical pulmonary rehabilitation: an introduction

M.D.L. Morgan

Department of
Respiratory Medicine
and Thoracic Surgery,
Glenfield Hospital,
Leicester

Practical Pulmonary Rehabilitation.
Edited by Mike Morgan and Sally Singh.
Published in 1997 by Chapman & Hall, London.
ISBN 0 412 61810 9.

Introduction

In spite of recent advances in medical therapy and improvements in health education, chronic lung disease has a serious impact on the individual and remains a major economic and social burden to the community. Chronic obstructive pulmonary disease (COPD) is the most important category of chronic disabling lung disease to affect the developed world. In the UK there are about 26 000 deaths per year from COPD and 240 000 hospital admissions (Strachan, 1995). It is also estimated that 24 million working days are lost each year, while the overall cost to the nation is probably unknown. While smoking rates decline in the developed world the long-term effects of the habit will continue to be felt for decades to come. In other parts of the world where cigarette smoking rates are increasing, future epidemics of COPD may threaten the economy of developing countries. While the obvious solution to this problem would be to reduce the prevalence of cigarette smoking, this may not be practical in the foreseeable future. Even if cigarette smoking ceased immediately, the effects would still be evident for many years to come. There are also a smaller number of respiratory conditions, such as chronic stable asthma, fibrosing alveolitis and chest-wall deformity, which leave patients with disability which cannot be improved by conventional medical treatment. The broad aim of pulmonary rehabilitation is to achieve an improvement in physical and social functioning over and above that achieved by ordinary medical treatment.

History

The concept of rehabilitation is well established in many branches of medicine and surgery. The aim of rehabilitation is to restore the individual to the fullest medical, mental, emotional, social and vocational potential of which he or she is capable. This process is enthusiastically practised in neurology, orthopaedics and cardiac medicine. In these examples the benefits in terms of improved physical functioning and self-confidence may be obvious. In the UK at least, the uptake of the principles of rehabilitation to respiratory medicine has been slow to develop. There may be several reasons for this lack of enthusiasm. The philosophy of medicine, particularly in Europe, centres on the individual doctor–patient relationship at the expense of the health team approach which is necessary for the purpose of rehabilitation. As a consequence, medical care for respiratory disease focuses strongly on the pharmacological reversal of impairment rather than the acceptance of disability and optimization of functional capacity.

*The development of
disability in chronic lung
disease*

By contrast, the practice in North America has been completely different. The benefits of exercise and nutrition were recognized as important factors in the treatment of tuberculosis over a century ago. More recently, in the consumer-driven health care industry, the client's desire for functional improvement is reflected in the large number of rehabilitation programmes which have become available over the last 30 years. The form and structure of these programmes have varied widely but there are many reports of the physical and economic benefits from different centres.

In the UK, the delivery of health care has not until recently been directed so positively by consumer demand. As a result, the pressure to provide rehabilitation programmes has not been very strong. In addition, the more objective scientific studies which have predominantly examined outcome measures of impairment have not demonstrated dramatic or prolonged benefit. These conditions have probably delayed the introduction of pulmonary rehabilitation programmes in the UK. Recently the National Health Service reforms have generated consumer pressure to develop a functional approach to the management of COPD. There have also been advances in the methods of assessment of physical performance and health-related quality of life which are more appropriate and sensitive to the improvements likely to be obtained through a successful programme. Alongside these changes there has also been a developing maturity in the scientific exploration of pulmonary rehabilitation with the reporting of genuine controlled studies which address some of the issues, while the National Institutes of Health in the USA have set the agenda for the future (Fishman, 1994). Following the success of clinical guidelines for asthma there has been interest in producing similar documents for COPD. The current guidelines clearly identify pulmonary rehabilitation as an important component of the medical care of COPD (Ferguson and Cherniak, 1993; American Thoracic Society, 1995; Siafakas *et al.*, 1995). A recent meta-analysis now clearly establishes the benefits of pulmonary rehabilitation programmes (Lacasse, 1996).

The development of disability in chronic lung disease

The development of lung disease is usually insidious and silent. Most chronic lung diseases such as COPD or pulmonary fibrosis develop slowly and may take decades before the damage results in noticeable symptoms. In a few conditions, such as asthma, the onset may be dramatic and result in immediate or intermittent disability. This contrasts with most other disciplines where the illness is sudden (e.g. stroke, accident or heart attack) and rehabilitation offers a road to recovery. This contrast does

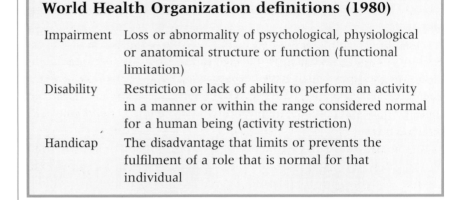

World Health Organization definitions (1980)

Impairment   Loss or abnormality of psychological, physiological or anatomical structure or function (functional limitation)

Disability   Restriction or lack of ability to perform an activity in a manner or within the range considered normal for a human being (activity restriction)

Handicap   The disadvantage that limits or prevents the fulfilment of a role that is normal for that individual

Box 1.1

Fig. 1.1 The effect of age and smoking on airway calibre (forced expiratory volume in 1 s; FEV$_1$). FEV$_1$ declines with age. Susceptible smokers decline more rapidly and develop symptoms in later life. Stopping smoking can return the rate of decline to that of non-smokers. After Fletcher and Peto (1977), with permission of the BMJ Publishing Group.

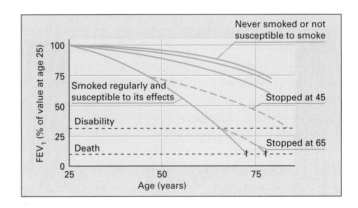

impose a slightly different philosophy upon pulmonary rehabilitation to the other similar disciplines. On the whole, chronic lung disease is progressive and unlikely to undergo spontaneous natural remission. Therefore the essence of rehabilitation in lung disease must begin with the premise that, once optimal medical treatment has been effected, the opportunities for improvement only exist through the reduction of disability rather than by the reversal of physical impairment. The distinction between the nature of impairment and the development of disability is fundamental to the appreciation of the benefits of pulmonary rehabilitation.

Impairment is defined as a reduction in strength or a weakness. In relation to lung disease, this means a reduction in physiological capacity resulting from pathological damage. Examples of impairment include a reduction in forced expiratory volume in 1 s (FEV$_1$) following airway damage in COPD, loss of respiratory muscle strength after polio or increased stiffness of the lungs in fibrosing alveolitis. In general, the pathological process has a predictable progressive effect upon impairment

(Fig. 1.1). For example, in the case of COPD, the decline in FEV_1 is directly related to survival (Fletcher and Peto, 1977; Pride and Burrows, 1995).

Disability is simply defined as the inability to perform a task or function as a result of impairment. In practice this may mean a reduction in exercise capacity leading to difficulty in carrying out simple routines which would normally be taken for granted. However it may have a more specific meaning in the context of exercise testing, e.g. endurance time or shuttle walk distance. It may also have a wider sociological inference when applied to the breakdown of social nexus or interaction. The relationship between impairment and disability is not as clear or predictable as that between pathology and impairment (Fig. 1.2).

Gradual impairment develops silently in lung disease since there is a reserve of functional capacity over requirement which is not needed in the lives of average people. For example, oxygen uptake and minute ventilation can increase by 15–20-fold at extremes of exercise but the majority of people in modern society seldom challenge these limits. Similarly, the respiratory muscle strength available to breathe exceeds that required to take an average breath by a factor of ten but is not required except in extreme circumstances. This large reserve of function can be eaten away by disease without any noticeable effect upon the lives of ordinary people. Furthermore, once symptoms do occur, it is relatively easy to modify lifestyle to avoid breathlessness by reducing activity. Lung disease may therefore progress for many years without any noticeable impact upon the life of the sufferer, who continues to compound the impairment by smoking. After approximately 60% of airway function is lost the symptoms of COPD cannot be disguised and the loss of function now starts to have an impact on everyday life. This is often perceived as a threshold of onset of the disease by the patient or doctor but actually

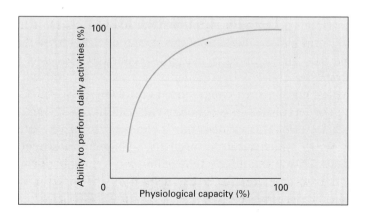

Fig. 1.2 Schematic representation of the relationship between loss of lung function (impairment) with disease and the effect on everyday activities (disability). Good function may be maintained until very late but the onset of disability may suddenly appear. By contrast, small improvements in function at a critical stage may produce a useful reduction in disability. After Jones (1988), with permission.

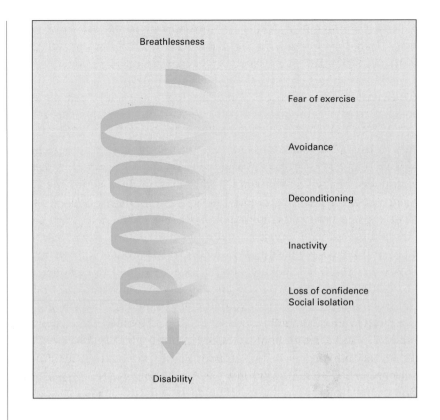

Breathlessness

Fear of exercise

Avoidance

Deconditioning

Inactivity

Loss of confidence
Social isolation

Disability

Fig. 1.3 The onset of
disability in lung disease is
compounded by inactivity and
loss of conditioning. Later this
inactivity will result in loss of
confidence and isolation.

reflects the continuing background development of impairment. The
exact level at which disability becomes significant is difficult to predict
from measures of impairment. Objective measures of exercise performance do not relate very well to individual indices of impairment such
as FEV_1, transfer factor for lung carbon monoxide (TLCO) or total lung
capacity (TLC) (Ortega *et al.*, 1994). The reasons for this are in part due
to the heterogeneous nature of pathology in COPD and also to the nature
of the development of disability in the later stages of illness (Fig. 1.3).

Most lung disease results in breathlessness which limits activity. The
degree to which dyspnoea prevents activity may be determined by the
individual threshold or tolerance of this symptom. This introduces a subjective but variable barrier to activity. The reduction of activity through
fear of dyspnoea and loss of confidence will result in reduced physical
fitness which may in turn compound the problem and lead to further
disability. On top of this, the disability can lead to loss of employment
and social isolation. This vicious cycle is characteristic of the later stages
of lung disease, which result in inactivity, isolation and dependence of
the sufferer. Since it is unlikely that pulmonary rehabilitation can alter
the fundamental impairment in lung disease it is evident that it has its

major effect in reducing disability by improving the factors which are not directly related to the initiating pathology but result from the multifactoral nature of decline of physical, psychological and social function.

Impairment, disability and handicap

As with other disabling conditions, the consequences of chronic lung disease have to be appreciated within their social context. The impact of disability will depend on the social and economic circumstances of the patient. For example, the handicap which results from a reduction in exercise capacity will be greater in people in manual employment than those with sedentary occupations. Similarly, the impact of disability will be harder in people who live alone than those who live with an active spouse who can drive a car. It is therefore important to consider the reduction of handicap rather than disability as the major target of rehabilitation. This will obviously require careful individual assessment and goal setting prior to rehabilitation to be most effective. To be comprehensive, the assessment should include recording of impairment (lung function), disability (exercise performance) and handicap (quality of life). Pulmonary rehabilitation may only have a significant effect upon disability and handicap once the impairment has been optimally addressed by medical treatment. A true functional approach to the management of COPD will require the correct assessment of each component and appreciation of the target of each intervention. For example, pharmacological treatment may improve impairment while exercise training can affect disability (Table 1.1).

Table 1.1 The functional management of chronic lung disease			
	Impairment	*Disability*	*Handicap*
	Damage	Reduced performance	Social impact
Assessment	Lung function	Exercise test	Quality of life questionnaire
Therapy	Steroids, bronchodilators, etc.	Exercise training	Education and psychosocial support

Definitions of pulmonary rehabilitation

In general, the culture of rehabilitation accepts that a major impairment is present which cannot be further improved by conventional medical treatment. Once this limitation is accepted, then the object of rehabilitation is to improve performance by the reduction of disability. This may involve treatments which are seemingly unconnected to the original illness. Rehabilitation is widely practised in other disciplines where the broad definition of rehabilitation is the restoration of the individual to the fullest medical, mental, emotional, social and vocational potential of which he or she is possible. It is difficult to challenge these aims as being irrelevant to lung disease but pulmonary rehabilitation has been slow to achieve acceptance, particularly in Europe where chronic lung disease remains a major burden. In North America, pulmonary rehabilitation has been embraced enthusiastically for the past two decades. Some of this enthusiasm may well have a commercial basis but there is also a pedigree of genuine scientific justification for its widespread application. To try to formalize pulmonary rehabilitation and to standardize programmes, the American College of Chest Physicians Committee on Pulmonary Rehabilitation adopted a definition in 1974. This was later endorsed by the American Thoracic Society and published as a statement in 1981. The definition is as follows:

> Pulmonary rehabilitation may be defined as an art of medical practice wherein an individually tailored, multidisciplinary program is formulated which through accurate diagnosis, therapy, emotional support, and education, stabilizes or reverses both the physio- and psychopathology of pulmonary diseases and attempts to return the patient to the highest possible functional capacity allowed by his pulmonary handicap and overall life situation.

This definition obviously has aesthetic defects but did usefully draw attention to the necessary components of rehabilitation and stress the prominence of individual prescription and multidisciplinary involvement. The definition has since been reviewed by a National Institutes of Health workshop (1994) in the light of the scientific development of the specialty to bring it up to date with the cultural perception of medicine as a science rather than an art. The current definition has been reformulated as:

> Pulmonary rehabilitation is a multidimensional continuum of services directed to persons with pulmonary disease and their families, usually by an interdisciplinary team of specialists, with the goal of achieving and maintaining the individual's maximum level of independence and functioning in the community.

Table 1.2 Comparison between the disciplines of respiratory and rehabilitation medicine

Respiratory medicine	Rehabilitation medicine
Strong doctor–patient relationship	Multidisciplinary team
Individual consultation	Group sessions
Long scientific pedigree	Recent scientific development
Many outcome measures	Few outcome measures
Little therapy	Lots of therapy

The same workshop also highlighted the historical contrasts between the philosophies of rehabilitation and respiratory medicine which may have dampened enthusiasm for rehabilitation in mainstream respiratory medicine. The recent history of medicine has been dominated by the development of the application of science to individual clinical skills. In respiratory medicine the background science has been predominantly physiology or, latterly, molecular biology and genetics. This combination of developments leads to a specialty which is centred around the doctor–patient relationship and has many outcome measures. By contrast, rehabilitation medicine has always been multidisciplinary and concentrates on therapy rather than measurement. This contrast partly explains the mutual separation of the disciplines (Table 1.2). Recent developments in the outcome measures to include more sensitive estimates of disability and quality of life mean that the scientific community may be more willing to appreciate the value of rehabilitation. At the same time the practitioners of rehabilitation are more sensitive to the need to express their results in scientific terms and also to analyse the process of rehabilitation to identify the optimum programme.

The process of rehabilitation

There is often some confusion in the world literature as to what activities constitute pulmonary rehabilitation. Many accounts include activities such as bronchodilator prescription which could reasonably be expected to form part of ordinary medical treatment. It is possible that in some centres rehabilitation provides access to specialist medical opinion that would otherwise be unavailable. There are also components of treatment such as oxygen therapy or ventilatory support which in

> # Categories of management of chronic obstructive pulmonary disease
>
> Prevention of further decline (e.g. smoking cessation)
>
> Reversing airflow obstruction (e.g. corticosteroids and bronchodilators)
>
> Supporting secondary pathophysiology (e.g. oxygen treatment)
>
> Optimizing functional capacity (e.g. rehabilitation)
>
> Surgical correction (e.g. transplant, bullectomy, lung volume reduction)

Box 1.2

some countries come under the auspices of the rehabilitation physician. For the purposes of this book we will properly consider pulmonary rehabilitation to be a definite separate clinical approach which assumes that all other medical aspects of treatment are optimally deployed. This approach is endorsed by the authors of guidelines on the management of COPD where pulmonary rehabilitation is identified as a separate modality from the treatment of airway obstruction or replacement oxygen or ventilatory support. The philosophy of pulmonary rehabilitation therefore accepts that residual disability exists and can be improved by techniques which do not primarily influence the underlying condition. Obviously, in the course of many rehabilitation programmes the acquisition of knowledge about medical treatment may improve its effectiveness, but this should be considered a byproduct of the process.

The components and structure of rehabilitation

There is some variation between centres in the interpretation of what constitutes pulmonary rehabilitation. Since rehabilitation is encouraged to be prescribed individually and delivered by different specialists, it is unlikely to be uniform. Furthermore, the availability of local skills will determine the spectrum of provision for each programme. Programmes with different components can be equally effective given common enthusiasm. The main components of pulmonary rehabilitation are contained in the three categories of exercise training, disease education and psychosocial support. The details of these components will be covered later in the book but the organization of the overall service requires some discussion.

The setting of pulmonary rehabilitation is not especially critical. Successful results have been described from inpatient, outpatient and

Components of pulmonary rehabilitation

Exercise training
Aerobic (brisk walking, cycling)
Strength
Respiratory muscle
Disease education
Pathology
Management
Physiotherapy
Relaxation
Coping skills
Drugs
Devices/oxygen
Smoking cessation
Sexual relations
Benefits and financial advice

Box 1.3

home-based programmes. The hospital-based outpatient programme is probably the most popular and efficient mode. Most of the skills required to set up and run a rehabilitation programme are available in the average hospital or community setting. The main contributors can include the respiratory physician, physiotherapist, occupational therapist, dietician, technician, nurse, social worker and even other patients. Usually, the contributions from these professionals are not very demanding and the call on their time may be easy to achieve, even in a busy hospital. It is, however, mandatory to identify at least one person to coordinate and plan the service. This role is often taken by the physiotherapist or respiratory nurse but this need not be exclusive. The duties of the coordinator will usually include planning the service, supervising exercise activities and producing literature. It is appropriate in larger programmes for this position to be a full-time or dedicated position but this may not always be necessary in smaller units. The coordinator will also be responsible for overseeing assessment, selection, evaluation and follow-up where applicable.

The processes of selection, assessment and evaluation are as important to the success of the overall programme as the rehabilitation process itself. Even where programmes may differ widely from each other in content, the basic assessments and outcome measures can be standardized. A formal selection procedure is important for several reasons. Assessment of the motivation of the patient may help preserve scarce resources and prevent drop-outs, which can have a dispiriting effect upon

Box 1.4

> ## Stages of pulmonary rehabilitation
>
> Referral
>
> Selection
>
> Assessment
>
> Rehabilitation
>
> Evaluation
>
> Maintenance and follow-up

groups. This can be achieved by psychological profiling or by informal interview. Usually the competition for places means that well-motivated subjects select themselves. The range of disability and age which can be considered is quite large, including those on oxygen therapy (Niederman *et al.*, 1991; Couser *et al.*, 1995). In those programmes which have cohort classes it is sensible to group people of similar ability together so that none are discouraged by the performance of others. Most programmes have a finite end or a graduation. In other countries it may be common to continue rehabilitation indefinitely, but this runs the risk of overloading the courses and encouraging dependence. It is also rather brutal to discharge patients at the end of a course, so some form of intermediate path such as physician review or self-help group such as Breathe Easy might be helpful.

Outcome measures

The philosophy of pulmonary rehabilitation, like rehabilitation in general, accepts that patients have an impairment of physiological capacity which may not be capable of correction. It seeks to develop those aspects of disability and social competence which can improve functional capacity. In the context of lung disease it is therefore unreasonable to expect improvements from rehabilitation in parameters of impairment such as FEV_1, blood gases or even maximal capacity. The outcome assessment of patients with chronic lung disease has to be more sophisticated and focused on function. In practice this means making an assessment of disability through an exercise test and some estimate of handicap through a quality of life measure. Disability is largely synonymous with exercise performance and can be assessed in the laboratory or the field. It is necessary in this context to distinguish between different types of exercise capacity which are relevant to patients' requirements. The measurement of maximal capacity may not reflect the functional activity of

*Evidence for the
effectiveness of pulmonary
rehabilitation*

a patient with lung disease and submaximal or endurance tests may be more appropriate. It is therefore important to match the assessment to the relevant activity. In the context of rehabilitation, exercise tests also have to be practical and possible to perform in a group setting. For this reason, field exercise tests of maximal capacity and walking endurance are more appropriate. The ideal global assessment of quality of life or handicap also does not exist. This is a developing field and there are now a number of general and disease-specific questionnaires which can be applied to the rehabilitation process to judge the effectiveness of the programmes. These measures have the same weaknesses as the exercise tests in so far that they do not necessarily cross-correlate and may examine different aspects of psychosocial behaviour.

Evidence for the effectiveness of pulmonary rehabilitation

The results of early rehabilitation programmes were often deemed to be disappointing because they did not seem to alter the course of the disease. There have also been few randomized controlled trials which have examined the outcome with any sensitivity. Much early research has been uncontrolled and observational and used outcome measures which we now appreciate may be insensitive to change. The more recent studies and reviews have greater scientific credibility and demonstrate that it is possible to achieve useful improvements in functional capacity and genuine health gain (Toshima *et al.*, 1990; Goldstein *et al.*, 1994; Celli, 1995; Morgan *et al.*, 1995; Ries *et al.*, 1995; Wijkstra *et al.*, 1996).

Mortality

Mortality in chronic lung disease, particulary COPD, is inversely related to FEV_1 and pulmonary rehabilitation would not expect to make much impact. There may be the occasional patient in whom a covert bronchodilator or steroid response has been uncovered during the programme. There are great difficulties in constructing a long-term randomized controlled trial to demonstrate the effect. Some studies have made comparisons with population controls and may show some small benefit of longevity. Comparisons of the survival curves of different programmes are heavily influenced by selection bias. However, increasing the length of life is not an aim of pulmonary rehabilitation. It is more important to improve the quality of life and independence in the remaining years.

There is also some evidence that patients who attend rehabilitation programmes would like to use the opportunity to define advanced directives regarding their terminal care (Heffner *et al.*, 1996).

Reduction of disability

As expected, pulmonary rehabilitation does not result in consistent improvements in static pulmonary function. Several randomized controlled studies have failed to demonstrate improvements in spirometry or gas exchange, in spite of demonstrable improvements in exercise capacity. One of the difficulties of appraising the results of rehabilitation is the inability to separate out the effects of the different elements with any confidence. However, the separate effects of exercise training on rehabilitation have been examined reasonably closely. These studies, predominantly with aerobic exercise, demonstrate that improvements can be achieved in walking test performance, submaximal testing and occasionally in maximal testing. However modest these improvements may seem, it is important to remember that even maintaining stability in these patients could be considered a success.

Other types of exercise training have also been studied. There appear to be useful benefits associated with strength-building and upper-body exercise. The position of inspiratory muscle training is less clear. It appears superficially to be an appropriate therapy but this is not supported by the available evidence. It appears that training for inspiratory muscle stength or endurance is task specific and the effect does not extend to improvements in whole-body performance or quality of life. It cannot therefore be recommended as a useful component, although it is suggested that it may augment the effect of aerobic cycle training (Wanke *et al.*, 1994). The application of exercise training and detailed results will be outlined in later chapters of the book.

Symptoms and quality of life

For the individual patient, the benefits of pulmonary rehabilitation will be the reduction in symptoms, improved functional capacity and independence in daily life. Recent evidence suggests that symptoms and subjective measures of dyspnoea are more closely related to functional ability than to conventional physiological parameters. The social consequences of deteriorating lung disease are also more important determinants of disability than the disturbance of physiology. Studies which demonstrate improvements in symptoms, coping skills, self-esteem or quality of life will therefore have important implications.

Pulmonary rehabilitation reduces the sensation of dyspnoea on exercise through desensitization or improved efficiency of exercise. It is not clear whether this is due to the effect of exercise training or a change in perception brought about by a reduction in anxiety or improvement in self-efficacy. It is likely that the patient can simply be desensitized to dyspnoea through the confidence of exercising under supervision (Reardon *et al.*, 1994). The improvements in quality of life measures appear to be consistently improved by most forms of pulmonary rehabilitation. Improvements have been demonstrated in dyspnoea scores, general health and disease-specific questionnaires. In fact, psychosocial intervention of any kind appears to have positive effects on social function, and intervention by rehabilitation or self-help groups may reduce the frequency of hospital admissions. The ease with which this improvement can be obtained does illustrate how easy it is to improve patients' lives simply by taking an interest. In some studies the psychological measures have improved in the control groups because they have been observed but without parallel change in performance.

Health gain and economic benefits

Chronic lung disease usually affects people in later life, resulting in increasing disability, dependence and frequency of hospital admissions. The effect of the disease is also felt by the family or carers and places an unknown burden on the community. The purpose of pulmonary rehabilitation is not to prolong life but to sustain independence and reduce health care expenditure. Obviously the evidence for this effectiveness has been obtained from the USA where the financial penalties for illness and hospital admission may be large. Pulmonary rehabilitation is recognized for reimbursement by insurers because published evidence illustrates that rehabilitation is effective in substantially reducing hospital admissions and other medical costs. Until recently there has been no motivation in the UK to reduce acute hospital admissions for COPD, but the National Health Service reforms may well stimulate a change in this attitude.

The cost of pulmonary rehabilitation will depend upon the type of service offered. Inpatient rehabilitation is obviously expensive and is rarely practised in the UK. However, it does appear that short-term outpatient or even community-based rehabilitation is equally effective. In all three modes, the beneficial effects can be present for at least 6 months and could be sustained by a minimum level of maintenance support.

After rehabilitation: the maintenance of benefit

Although pulmonary rehabilitation does not necessarily offer a survival advantage for patients with lung disease, it does apparently improve the quality of their remaining lives. By inference, this is also likely to improve

Box 1.5

Maintenance of benefit

Continued rehabilitation

Infrequent refresher sessions

Spot reviews

Telephone support

Training diaries and exercise manual

Self-help groups

the quality of the lives of carers and other family members. The benefits of rehabilitation, once they are achieved, appear to be long-lasting. However, it is reasonable to assume that some sort of maintenance of benefit can be prolonged by aftercare. Obviously, the rehabilitation programme could be continued indefinitely but this expensive support would be contrary to the philosophy of self-efficacy that is promoted during the initial programme. There are several low-cost alternatives to continued attendance at classes which may be able to sustain improvement but there is very little research in this area.

The development of self-help groups is a particularly attractive option in the UK. The Breathe Easy support groups are growing in number as members recognize the benefits. These type of support groups are more likely to succeed in patients with chronic lung disease than in younger patients with, for example, asthma or diabetes where the natural tendency is to shrug off the condition. Regular meetings with fellow sufferers and spouses offer the opportunity for mutual support and encouragement to maintain activity. Groups may also maintain telephone contact and offer support for colleagues who are unable to attend the meetings. The content of the meetings, which is determined by the group, is usually related to education about some aspect of lung disease and its management. The important feature is that members of the group now feel that they are less dependent and are in control of some aspects of their lives. Contribution to an active group or participation in fund-raising events may provide a purpose to life which has been missing for years.

References

American Thoracic Society. (1981) Pulmonary rehabilitation. *Am. Rev. Respir. Dis.* **124**:663–6.

American Thoracic Society. (1995) Standards for the diagnosis and care of patients with chronic obstructive pulmonary disease. *Am. J. Respir. Crit. Care Med.* **152**:s77–120.

Celli, B.R. (1995) Pulmonary rehabilitation in patients with COPD. *Am. J. Respir. Crit. Care Med.* **152**:861–4.

Couser, J.I., Guthmann, R., Hamadeh, M.A., and Kane, C.S. (1995) Pulmonary rehabilitation improves exercise capacity in older elderly patients with COPD. *Chest* **107**:730–4.

Ferguson, G.T., and Cherniak, R.M. (1993) Management of chronic obstructive pulmonary disease. *N. Engl. J. Med.* **128**:1017–22.

Fishman, A.P. (1994) Pulmonary rehabilitation research. *Am. J. Respir. Crit. Care Med.* **149**:825–33.

Fletcher, C., and Peto, R. (1977) The natural history of chronic airflow obstruction. *Br. Med. J.* **1**:1645–8.

Goldstein, R.S., Gort, E.H., Stubbing, D. *et al.* (1994) Randomised controlled trial of respiratory rehabilitation. *Lancet* **344**:1394–7.

Heffner, J.E., Fahy, B., Hilling, L. (1996) Activities regarding advanced directives among patients in pulmonary rehabilitation. *Am. J. Respir. Crit. Care Med.* **154**:1735–40.

Jones, N.L. (1988) *Clinical Exercise Testing*, 3rd edn. Philadelphia: WB Saunders.

Lacasse, Y., Wong, E., Guyatt, G.H. *et al.* (1996) Meta-analysis of respiratory rehabilitation in chronic obstructive pulmonary disease. *Lancet* **348**:1115–89.

Morgan, M.D.L., Quirk, F.H., Singh, S.J. (1995) Purchasing for quality–pulmonary rehabilitation. *Quality in Health Care* **4**:284–8.

National Institutes of Health workshop summary. (1994) Pulmonary rehabilitation research. *Am. J. Respir. Crit. Care Med.* **149**:825–33.

Niederman, M.S., Clemente, P.H., Fein, A.M., *et al.* (1991) Benefits of a multidisciplinary pulmonary rehabilitation programme. *Chest* **99**:798–804.

Ortega, F., Montemayor, T., Sanchez, A., *et al.* (1994) The role of cardiopulmonary exercise testing and the criteria used to determine disability in patients with severe chronic obstructive lung disease. *Am. J. Respir. Crit. Care Med.* **150**:747–51.

Pride, N.B., Burrows, B. (1995) Development of impaired lung function. In: *Chronic Obstructive Pulmonary Disease* (eds P.M.A. Calverley and N.B. Pride). London: Chapman & Hall, pp. 69–91.

Reardon, J., Awad, E., Normandin, E. *et al.* (1994) The effect of comprehensive outpatient pulmonary rehabilitation on dyspnoea. *Chest* **105**:1046–52.

Ries, A.L., Kaplan, R.M., Limberg, T.M., Prewitt, L.M. (1995) Effects of pulmonary rehabilitation on physiologic and psychosocial outcomes in patients with chronic obstructive pulmonary disease. *Ann. Intern. Med.* **122**:823–32.

Siafakas, N.M., Vermeire, P., Pride, N.B. *et al.* (1995) Optimal assessment and management of chronic obstructive pulmonary disease. *Eur. Respir. J.* **8**:1398–1420.

Strachan, D.A. (1995) Epidemiology: a British perspective. In: *Chronic Obstructive Pulmonary Disease* (eds P.M.A. Calverley and N.B. Pride). London: Chapman & Hall, pp. 47–67.

Toshima, M.T., Kaplan, R.M., Ries, A.L. (1990) Experimental evaluation of rehabilitation in chronic obstructive pulmonary disease: short term effects on exercise endurance and health status. *Health Psychol.* **9**:237–52.

Wanke, T., Formanek, D., Lahrman, H. *et al.* (1994) Effects of combined inspiratory muscle and cycle ergometer training on exercise performance in patients with COPD. *Eur. Respir. J.* **7**:2205–11.

Wijkstra, P.J., van der Mark, Th.W., Kraan, J. *et al.* (1996) Effects of home rehabilitation on physical performance in patients with chronic obstructive pulmonary disease. *Eur. Respir. J.* **9**:104–10.

World Health Organization (WHO). (1980) *International Classification of Impairments, Disabilities, and Handicaps.* Geneva: WHO.

2. Patient selection and assessment for pulmonary rehabilitation

S.J. Singh

Department of
Respiratory Medicine
and Thoracic Surgery,
Glenfield Hospital,
Leicester

Practical Pulmonary Rehabilitation.
Edited by Mike Morgan and Sally Singh.
Published in 1997 by Chapman & Hall, London.
ISBN 0 412 61810 9.

Introduction

Patient selection is one of the most important considerations when starting a rehabilitation programme. The inappropriate identification of patients most likely to benefit from the course can prejudice the success of the programme. Inevitably, a variety of opinions exist to identify the optimal client group to target for rehabilitation. However, the application of purely clinical criteria is complicated by fundamental considerations such as patient motivation and travel difficulties. This chapter will address these and other issues when selecting patients for pulmonary rehabilitation together with some of the more important aspects of patient assessment.

At present in the UK the majority of organized rehabilitation services are outpatient based. Commonly in the UK, candidates for pulmonary rehabilitation are processed within the hospital, although some centres are exploring the feasibility of offering home- and community-based programmes. These options have been explored more extensively in Europe (Wijkstra *et al.*, 1995).

Why refer for pulmonary rehabilitation?

Acknowledgment by the individual (or close relative or friend) of a decline in physical performance is a prerequisite for rehabilitation. This insidious loss of fitness results in the individual adopting a less demanding lifestyle and, as frequently described throughout this text, the individual becomes trapped in a vicious circle of inactivity, breathlessness, depression and social isolation. A crude evaluation of the individual's decreasing physical ability is to enquire if he or she can keep up with a friend or relative of the same age whilst out walking.

Additional reasons for referral might include a disproportionate level of disability in relation to the level of impairment or a loss of confidence in performing physical activity. Less commonly, patients are referred for dietary advice in conjunction with an exercise programme or for control of abnormal breathing patterns.

Which patients to refer?

The team accepting the referral for pulmonary rehabilitation assumes that the individual has been thoroughly assessed and managed by the referring specialist or general practitioner to such a degree that no further gains can be achieved by additional pharmaceutical intervention, and

Patient selection

Chronic obstructive pulmonary disease

Clinically stable

Optimal pharmaceutical management

Declining functional capacity

No coexistent neurological or orthopaedic problem (to inhibit mobility)

Motivated

Smokers (i.e. programme to take a view on this)

Box 2.1

second, that the decreased physical fitness and associated dyspnoea are related to a respiratory pathology and not, for example, as a consequence of a cardiac abnormality.

Most commonly, patients are referred with a diagnosis of chronic obstructive pulmonary disease (COPD), ideally during a period of clinical stability. This group of patients has traditionally been categorized into mild, moderate or severe, employing the criteria laid down by the American Thoracic Society using spirometry (1987). Examining the literature, there are no guidelines on the category of patients to accept. Various authors provide evidence that rehabilitation is appropriate for a wide range of patients with COPD, including those severely impaired and disabled (Sinclair and Ingram, 1977; Tydeman *et al.*, 1984; Casaburi *et al.*, 1991). It is documented elsewhere in this text that lung function relates poorly to exercise tolerance, therefore basing selection upon lung function alone is inherently unsound.

Patients with respiratory disease other than COPD

Patients with alternative (non-COPD) respiratory pathologies have been incorporated into a rehabilitation programme with promising results (The Toronto Lung Transplant Group, 1988; Foster and Thomas, 1990). Patients for consideration could include those with:

- Bronchiectasis.
- Disorders of the thoracic spine (ankylosing spondylitis; thoracoplasty, following tuberculosis).
- Scoliosis, kyphoscoliosis, e.g. congenital or secondary to polio.
- Recovering chest trauma.
- Pre and post lung resection.

■ Pre and post lung transplantation.
■ Pre and post volume reduction surgery.

Preliminary research suggests that rehabilitation may be worthwhile prior to volume reduction surgery (Cooper *et al.*, 1995). Inevitably, it is difficult to suggest which group may be most worthwhile targeting. From our own experience it appears that the magnitude of the improvement in terms of exercise tolerance for non-COPD patients (for example, kyphoscoliosis and fibrosing alveolitis) is comparable to patients with COPD.

Which patients to consider with care?

The structure of a pulmonary rehabilitation programme, regardless of its location, is reasonably consistent – an educational and exercise component, with a large percentage of patients benefiting from both components. In view of the age of this population it is likely that there will be coexisting abnormalities. Patients should not be denied rehabilitation because of this. However, patients who present with a limitation to exercise not linked with the respiratory system (e.g. coexisting locomotor, neurological or cardiovascular pathologies) are unlikely to respond to aerobic training. Clearly, the limitation to exercise must be defined. If it subsequently appears that the cause is not linked to the respiratory system, the patient can be invited to the education component of the programme, discussed in detail throughout the book.

Individuals should not be discriminated against because of their age (Ambrosino and Foglio, 1996), disease severity or sex. But if their particular circumstances dictate, it may be necessary to defer recruitment to the programme until the cohort is more compatible. This is most apparent when the individual requires supplemental oxygen.

As previously stated, patients considered for rehabilitation should be established on their medication and clinically stable. Patients who have been referred whilst on the ward should be assessed for pulmonary rehabilitation following a satisfactory outpatient follow-up. Occasionally, it may be necessary to accept a person during the convalescent phase of an exacerbation; this is particularly relevant for patients who have frequent admissions.

A final point in this section is the selection of patients who currently smoke. Some centres will not accept current smokers until they can demonstrate a reasonable period of abstention. Others will accept the smoker and offer practical help and advice to stop. It is the opinion of some that patients who cannot refrain from smoking are unlikely to comply with a rehabilitation programme and embrace lifestyle changes.

It is probable that in any cohort a majority will be ex-smokers, but having stopped smoking successfully they can both empathize and encourage current smokers to quit. It may be worth considering setting up a small 'stop smoking' self-help group within the hospital. This service is commonly led by a nurse from the respiratory wards. To encourage patients to stop smoking a variety of techniques can be offered to smooth the transition from smoker to non-smoker.

Which patients to exclude?

Overall there are few patients with a diagnosis of chronic obstructive lung disease who would not benefit from either component of a pulmonary rehabilitation course. However, a few exceptions need to be recognized:

- Patients not motivated to attend regularly.
- Patients not committed to instigate lifestyle changes.
- Those with travel difficulties.
- Those with work difficulties (either difficulties with time off for attendance or requiring an out-of-hours programme).
- Those with language difficulties. In inner-city areas with a substantial immigrant population problems with language may be overcome by using an interpreter (either an official or a relative).

Hearing problems are usually easily overcome. A barrier less easily overcome is for those patients presenting with an unstable psychiatric history.

Can oxygen-dependent patients be included?

Patients requiring oxygen therapy need not be excluded from a rehabilitation programme. It is important that these patients are carefully assessed to evaluate their requirements for ambulatory oxygen during the exercise session. It is worthwhile having a group where at least a couple of patients use oxygen to overcome embarrassment or self-consciousness. Figure 2.1 summarizes a possible mechanism for patient selection.

Assessment for pulmonary rehabilitation

There are five main objectives of the assessment:

1. Evaluate the magnitude of the signs and symptoms (the level of impairment).
2. Quantify exercise tolerance (the level of disability).

Patient selection and
assessment for pulmonary
rehabilitation

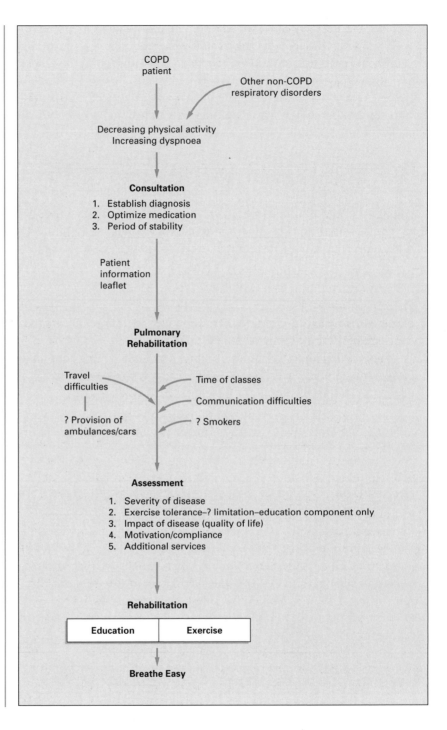

Fig. 2.1 A guide to patient selection for pulmonary rehabilitation. COPD = chronic obstructive pulmonary disease.

3. Assess the impact of the disease on the individual's day-to-day life (including quality of life – the handicap).
4. Identify those individuals likely to graduate from a programme (including goal setting).
5. Identify those individuals requiring additional individual treatment from the professionals represented in the team.

The culmination of these objectives is to ensure that pulmonary rehabilitation offers an effective treatment.

The assessment presents an ideal opportunity to become familiar with the patient and partner and their expectations of pulmonary rehabilitation. Ideally, the patient and partner should communicate a desire to improve the patient's quality of life and express some commitment to and enthusiasm for a course of pulmonary rehabilitation. The information from the partner, on the one hand, can corroborate the severity of the disease symptoms expressed by the patient or, alternatively, conflict with the patient's account of functional impairment, frequency and severity of symptoms. Nevertheless, information from the spouse is useful and his or her support for the programme can increase patient compliance and adherence to the regimen.

Evaluation of the magnitude of the signs and symptoms

Objective measures of the magnitude of impairment are discussed in Chapter 8. Access to medical records will confirm the severity, duration and course of disease (usually with measures of lung function and arterial blood-gas analysis), concurrent disease and medication. The information from the records identifies the level of impairment and secures an accurate evaluation of the individual.

The basic data required are summarized in Table 2.1. The information collected is broadly divided into two categories: physiological and psychological. The physiological data (resting and during exercise) allow an estimation of impairment and disability. The psychological component reflects, in part, the level of handicap and emotional status and the impact that the respiratory disease has on the patient's everyday life. The auditing of the number of days in hospital, hospital consultations and visits to the general practitioner allows a meaningful evaluation of the demand upon health care resources.

The resting physiological measurements are summarized in Table 2.2. Heart rate can either be measured directly or during exercise with a short-range telemetry device (Fig. 2.2). Such a device allows the continual monitoring of heart rate during exercise. This type of monitor, recording rate not rhythm, does give some warning of cardiovascular problems if the resting heart rate or response to exercise is inappropriate.

Table 2.1 Basic data required at initial assessment
Date . . . .
Name . . . .
Address . . . .
Telephone . . . .
Specialist . . . .
General practitioner . . . .
Date of birth/age . . . .
Civil status . . . .
Housing . . . .
Occupation . . . .
Retired/disability/redundant . . .
Hobbies . . . .
Main diagnosis . . . .
Concurrent diagnosis . . . .
Medication . . . .
Inhaled . . . .
Inhaler technique satisfactory: yes/no
Nebulized . . . .
Requires spacer/volumatic yes/no
Other . . . .
Oxygen . . . .
Requirement p.r.n./long-term oxygen therapy
Number of days in hospital due to respiratory problem
. . . .
Number of hospital consultations
. . . .
Number of courses of antibiotics
. . . .
Number of courses of steroids
. . . .

ASSESSMENT OF GAS EXCHANGE

An impairment in the efficiency of the lungs to deliver oxygen or eliminate carbon dioxide may become apparent when analysing a sample of arterial blood. Patients with severe COPD demonstrate hypoxaemia and,

Table 2.2 An example of the resting physiological data to be collected

Heart rate . . . .

Respiratory rate . . . .

Blood pressure . . . .

Oxygen saturation . . . .

FEV_1 . . . .

Predicted . . . .

FVC . . . .

FEV/FEV_1 (%) . . . .

Breathlessness . . . .

FEV_1 = Forced expiratory volume in 1 s; FVC = forced vital capacity; FEV = forced expiratory volume.

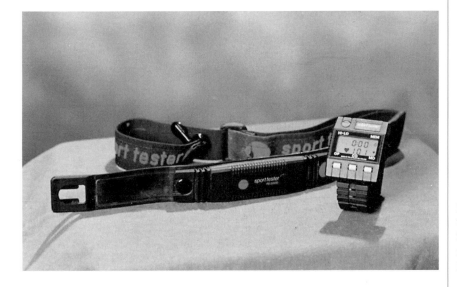

Fig. 2.2 A short-range telemetry device that is used to monitor ambulatory heart rate (sports tester PE3000; Polar).

with increasing severity of the disease, hypercapnia. (Normal ranges for the partial pressure of arterial oxygen (PaO$_2$) and carbon dioxide (PaCO$_2$) are 12–14 and 4.5–6.5 kPa respectively.)

There is a link between the reduction in the forced expiratory volume in 1s (FEV_1) and declining PaO$_2$. The PaCO$_2$ may remain within normal limits until the FEV_1 falls below 1.2–1.5 l (Snider *et al.*, 1994). Oxygen saturation can be measured by a portable pulse oximeter. This should be measured at rest and during exercise. The relationship between measurements of oxygen saturation and arterial blood gases may not always correlate as well as anticipated, because of a variety of technical and physiological mechanisms. At rest, oxygen saturation should be above 94% in a healthy individual; any value below 85% requires a blood sample to be taken for analysis to confirm hypoxaemia. If this is confirmed, the patient should be referred back to the consultant or general practitioner for consideration of continuous supplemental oxygen therapy.

ASSESSMENT OF BREATHLESSNESS

Breathlessness/dyspnoea can be defined as 'an awareness of the act of breathing, usually occurring when ventilation or the effort required to ventilate the lungs is excessive' (Howell, 1990), or alternatively, 'occurring when the demand for ventilation exceeds the patient's ability to respond' (West, 1987). The feeling of breathlessness can manifest itself to the patient in a variety of ways: the patient may complain of chest tightness, an inability to fill the lungs or simply, difficulty in breathing. The feeling is personal assessment and not a physical phenomenon that can be quantified objectively (Sweer and Zwillich, 1990). There is no one simple explanation of the cause of dyspnoea; however, a number of contributing factors have been suggested. A variety of signals may be responsible for mediating the sensation of breathlessness, including the chemoreceptors in the blood and brain, mechanoreceptors in the thorax and outgoing central nervous system respiratory motor commands (Altose, 1985).

An increase in the ventilatory drive is produced by hypoxaemia, hypercapnia, acidaemia and exercise in patients with COPD. Both hypoxaemia and hypercapnia evoke the sensation of dyspnoea but produce shortness of breath via different mechanisms – the stimulation of the carotid bodies in hypoxic patients and via direct stimulation of the brainstem in patients with a high $PaCO_2$. Swinburn *et al.* (1984) demonstrated the effect of hypoxia on breathlessness in patients with COPD. They found that the administration of oxygen during exercise prevented the previous falls in oxygen saturation and also improved breathlessness.

For patients with COPD the abnormal sensation of breathlessness is multifactorial. The predominant factor is thought to be related to hyperinflation of the lungs (Howell, 1990) and the influence this has upon the respiratory muscles (Sweer and Zwillich, 1990). Lung hyperinflation results in the diaphragm being flatter than normal and therefore forced to operate within a non-optimal portion of the length–tension curve, like the inspiratory muscles. In the normal lung the optimal position for

> ## Assessment of dyspnoea
>
> *Functional impairment*
> Medical Research Council breathlessness scale
> Oxygen cost diagram
> Mahler dyspnoea index
> Dyspnoea component of Chronic Respiratory Disease
> Questionnaire
> *Symptom intensity*
> Visual analogue score
> Borg breathlessness score
> Borg perceived exertion
> *Physiological measures*
> Dyspnoea index

Box 2.2

diaphragm contraction is at functional residual capacity (FRC) but in COPD the muscle is shortened and requires a greater motor input to evoke a satisfactory shortening (Rochester, 1991). The actual configuration of the diaphragm is altered; normally, the diaphragm increases in both the transverse and anteroposterior diameters of the chest when contracting, but in the hyperinflated chest the lower ribs may in fact be drawn in (Howell, 1990). In an attempt to relieve dyspnoea a patient will spontaneously lean forwards. In doing so the diaphragm is pushed proximally into a more efficient position.

The assessment of dyspnoea is difficult, not least because it is something that the patient feels, it is affected by both emotional and environmental factors and it cannot be measured accurately. An easily applied scale is required that can reveal either the functional impairment experienced as a result of the breathlessness or the magnitude of the sensation associated with a particular activity. There are just a handful of scales available. To quantify the functional impairment the Medical Research Council (MRC) breathlessness scale (1966), the oxygen cost diagram (McGavin *et al.*, 1978) and the Mahler baseline and transitional dyspnoea index (Mahler *et al.*, 1984) can be used. The first scale requires patients to choose a verbal description of their sensation of breathlessness and the associated functional limitations. The descriptions are divided into categories, for example (using the MRC scale), the patient may choose from one of five options (e.g. number 3: patient walks slower than most people on the level). The oxygen cost diagram requires patients to mark on a vertical 10-cm line the level corresponding to the point where their breathlessness would not allow them to continue. Alongside this line is a list of daily activities. The Mahler dyspnoea index and transitional index allow individuals to rate their dyspnoea and from this, identify changes from the baseline value. Rating of the dyspnoea has three categories: functional impairment, magnitude of the task and magnitude of effort. Until a modification by Stoller *et al.* (1986), the functional impairment was confined to limitations associated with work; the scale now allows for impairments either at home or work to be scored.

An alternative to rating functional disability is to rate the intensity of the symptoms associated with a particular activity. The two scales most commonly used are the visual analogue score (VAS) and the Borg score (Borg, 1982). The VAS comprises a 10-cm line labelled from 0 to 10 with descriptors of nothing to maximal at either end. Patients mark along the line the intensity of the sensation. For this method the stimulus–response is treated in a linear fashion (Jones, 1988) and the patient effectively assigns a numerical value to a sensation.

There are two Borg scores; both are used in the assessment of patients with COPD. The original scale of perceived exertion has numerical values from 6 to 20 with descriptors (very, very light to very, very hard) placed against seven numbers on the scale. The modified Borg scale (1982) is used to assess patients' perceived breathlessness in response to an intervention, commonly exercise. The adjectives range from 'nothing at all' to 'maximal' and are assigned a value ranging from 0 to 10. Borg (1982) proposed that the scale allows an interindividual comparison to be made. The category scale increases linearly as exercise intensity increases and is closely correlated to physiological responses that also increase linearly, such as heart rate (American College of Sports Medicine, 1991). It is suggested that the position of the descriptors is such that a doubling of the numerical rating corresponds to a similar increase in the intensity of the sensation. Because of their simplicity, both the VAS and Borg scores allow the assessment of breathlessness during activity.

A more objective approach to define dyspnoea is to relate exercise ventilation to a maximal voluntary ventilation (MVV). This ratio, $V_{E_{max}}/MVV$, where $V_{E_{max}}$ = maximum ventilation, was termed the dyspnoea index. More recently, this relationship has been used to describe the ventilatory reserve during exercise rather than dyspnoea (Clark, 1991).

Dyspnoea ratings   A resting measure of breathlessness allows the assessor to identify the individual with an inappropriately high or low level of breathlessness as well as judge exercise dyspnoea in relation to baseline dyspnoea. A small reported rest to exercise change can identify patients who:

- Have a fear of being breathless.
- Overestimated their resting levels.
- Underestimated their exercise level.

■ Tolerate exercise not limited by dyspnoea.
■ Are anxious.
■ Have a desire to underperform to establish the severity of their disease.

Whatever the reason, it is important to observe the patient's behaviour, symptoms and recovery time.

Assessment of exercise tolerance

Lung function tests (e.g. FEV_1 and forced vital capacity) do not relate well to a patient's functional capacity. Most studies reveal a poor relationship between the two (McGavin *et al.*, 1978; Swinburn *et al.*, 1985). Consequently, exercise tests are employed to evaluate more precisely a patient's level of disability and ability to perform day-to-day activities. In terms of pulmonary rehabilitation, an exercise test is not only useful to quantify the individual's exercise tolerance but also is important as an indicator of change. Rehabilitation, not surprisingly, has no effect upon lung function (Simpson *et al.*, 1992). Furthermore, an exercise test is important prior to entry to a rehabilitation programme to indicate the limitations to exercise – respiratory, peripheral or cardiovascular. If the individual fails to continue with an exercise test because of breathlessness it is likely that the respiratory system is the limitation to exercise. Alternatively, if the patient stops because of general fatigue it is likely that he or she is deconditioned and will respond to exercise training. If, however, the test is aborted because of cardiovascular reasons, leg pain, intermittent claudication, angina, etc., it is unlikely that he or she will respond to exercise training within the context of pulmonary rehabilitation. It is vitally important to make this distinction. Patients presenting with a coexisting history of osteoarthritis or angina are not uncommon, but this may *not* be a limiting factor to exercise.

Two environments for testing exist – formal laboratory assessment and, more commonly, field tests. In each, a wealth of protocols exist (Fig. 2.3), with options including unpaced, unstructured, incremental and

---

Why use an exercise test?

To identify functional abnormalities not present at rest

To identify the true extent of the limitation

To monitor levels of oxygen saturation

As an aid in differential diagnosis for limitation to exercise

To prescribe an exercise programme

To evaluate the response to rehabilitation

Box 2.3

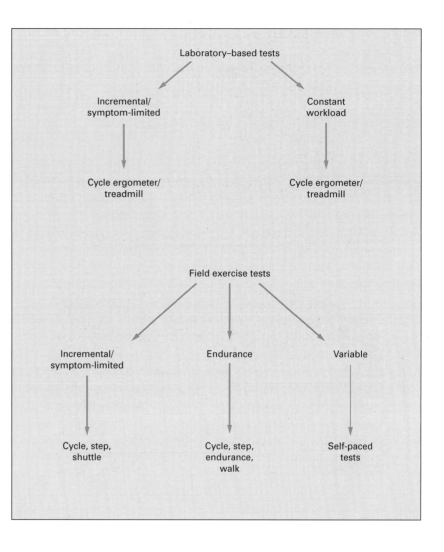

Fig. 2.3 Exercise tests employed to assess cardiorespiratory capacity in patients with chronic obstructive pulmonary disease.

maximal. Laboratory assessment requires patients to perform a treadmill or cycle ergometer test; with detailed gas analysis measurements the patient wears either a face mask or mouthpiece and nose clips (Fig. 2.4). This form of testing is not widely available, being confined to larger centres where the technical support exists. Moreover, the equipment (treadmill and gas analysis equipment) is expensive and the procedures involved quite intimidating to the patient. Consequently, field exercise tests were developed as a cheap, simple and effective alternative to laboratory-based assessment of disability. Field tests of walking ability are most frequently employed. The most familiar tests are self-paced tests where the patient is required to walk as far as possible in either 12 or 6 min (McGavin *et al.*, 1976; Butland *et al.*, 1982). These protocols are difficult to standardize and may be overly influenced by motivation and

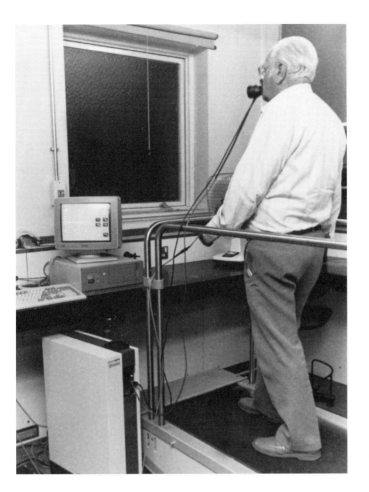

Fig. 2.4 Patient performing a laboratory-based exercise test: (a) treadmill walking test.

encouragement. In addition, their simplicity limits the information which can be obtained from them about the physiological and symptomatic changes occurring during exercise. More recently, the shuttle walking test has been developed as a standardized field exercise test (Singh *et al.*, 1992) that is both reliable and valid (Fig. 2.5). The shuttle walking test is an incremental, externally paced exercise test that stresses the patient to a symptom-limited maximum. Briefly, the test requires the individual to walk around a 10-m course, defined by two marker cones. The speed of walking is dictated by signals played from a tape cassette and increases every minute until the patient is either too breathless to continue or cannot maintain the required speed. Because the speed of walking is externally controlled, the influence of the operator and/or encouragement is dampened. To improve the sensitivity of the test, measures of dyspnoea, exertion, oximetry and heart rate can be incorporated. However, a more specific diagnosis can only be made with laboratory testing.

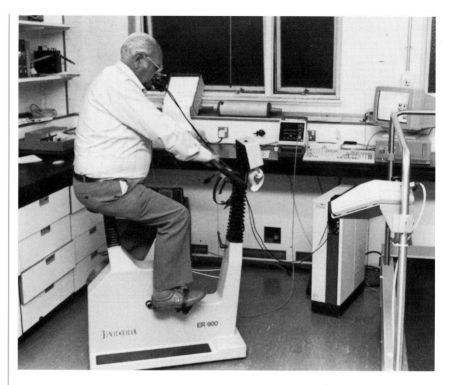

Fig. 2.4 Patient performing a laboratory-based exercise test: (b) cycle ergometer test.

Box 2.4

Adjuncts to field walking tests

Heart rate monitors
Oxygen saturation monitors
Dyspnoea ratings
Exertion ratings
Portable oxygen consumption meters
Blood lactate concentrations

If space is at an absolute premium, a step test would allow an objective assessment of exercise, providing that a metronome was available to facilitate a range of constant and/or incremental protocols. The disadvantage of step tests is the difficulty associated in calculating the amount of work performed. Jones (1988) suggests that it is difficult to measure the power because of the difficulty in gauging the work done in stepping down. For patients who do not regularly climb stairs peripheral muscular fatigue, rather than a symptom of respiratory disease, may decrease performance. Both walking and step tests represent a form of exercise testing that can be performed outside the laboratory environment.

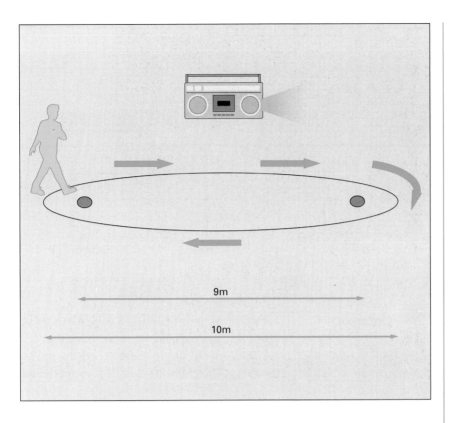

Fig. 2.5 The shuttle walking
test.

The most rigorous measure of exercise capacity is to measure directly
maximal oxygen uptake ($V_{O_{2max}}$; Astrand and Rodahl, 1986). In patients
with respiratory disorders the oxygen consumption (V_{O_2}) is limited due
to ventilatory abnormalities and consequently the maximal V_{O_2} a patient
attains is often described as the symptom-limited $V_{O_{2max}}$ or peak oxygen
consumption ($V_{O_{2peak}}$). A $V_{O_{2max}}$ is traditionally defined as the point at
which, despite an increase in the gradient or speed of the treadmill, there
is no accompanying increase in oxygen uptake (less than 150 ml
oxygen/min) – a plateau effect. This point is seldom achieved in patients
with COPD. For patients with COPD the limitation to exercise is due to
the inability of the lungs to meet the demand for increasing ventilation.
In healthy trained subjects the limit to continued exercise is the cardiovascular system – more specifically, the stroke volume.

There is a paucity of data relating existing field test performance to
$V_{O_{2peak}}$ in patients and consequently their validity in assessing exercise
tolerance must be questioned. A moderate relationship between the two
variables – distance walked versus $V_{O_{2max}}$ – was demonstrated for the 12-
min walking test. Recent work has revealed that the shuttle walking test
relates well to $V_{O_{2peak}}$ (Singh *et al.*, 1994). This direct relationship facilitates prescription of exercise, particularly endurance walking.

35

> # Treadmill versus cycle ergometer
>
> Treadmill takes up a lot of space
> Treadmill offers a familiar activity
> Cycle ergometer allows precise definition of workload
> Other physiological measures are easier with the cycle ergometer

Considerably more data are available examining patients' exercise tolerance in the laboratory environment, observing the ventilatory and physiological responses to exercise. The most commonly observed are $V_{O_{2peak}}$, carbon dioxide production (V_{CO_2}), V_E and heart rate. Less commonly identified are the V_{CO_2}/V_{O_2} and V_E/V_{O_2} slope, and blood lactate concentration. The latter is used in sophisticated rehabilitation programmes to identify a lactate threshold, and thus a training threshold. It is suggested that it is only those individuals reaching this threshold level that are able to induce physiological changes as a result of training. Progressive exercise tests can be performed on either a cycle ergometer or treadmill. The $V_{O_{2max}}$ reached for a healthy population during this form of exercise can be up to 10% lower on a cycle compared to that obtained during treadmill walking (Astrand and Rodahl, 1986). This discrepancy may not be consistently observed in COPD (Mathur *et al.*, 1995).

Tests of both maximal and submaximal exercise tolerance have their place in pulmonary rehabilitation. Once the maximal performance has been clearly established, the endurance (submaximal) capacity can be identified. The endurance test will reflect the ability to sustain a level of exercise at, for example, 50–60% of the $V_{O_{2peak}}$. In a healthy population it may be possible to extrapolate the V_{O_2}/heart rate slope to approximate the maximal work rate achievable. Alternatively, a predicted $V_{O_{2max}}$ can be calculated from some basic resting physiological measures:

85.42–13.75 (male 1, female 2) −0.409 age −3.24
(1 active, 2 sedentary) −0.114 (weight, kg)

(Bruce *et al.*, 1973). From this point a training regime can be prescribed at the desired level. Unfortunately, the linear relationship between work rate ($V_{O_{2peak}}$) and heart rate is not preserved in patients with COPD, making it difficult to prescribe exercise from a submaximal test.

Recently it has been proposed that the endurance test may be a more sensitive measure of improvement in exercise tolerance as a result of exercise training. This relates to the nature of the limitation in this group of patients. If the limit to exercise is truly a failure of the respiratory system to sustain the levels of ventilation required, then rehabilitation will not alter those parameters and it is likely that improvements in maximal exercise will be minimal. In the laboratory, endurance testing is straightforward but in the field, endurance testing is inevitably less precise where a step test or a walking test can be used. A constant-rate step test would be easier to calibrate than a walking test. A field endurance walk has been described in which the subject is instructed to walk as far as possible (at a pace as though late for an appointment) and to stop when unable to go any further (Davidson *et al.*, 1988). Maintenance of a constant prescribed speed of walking is obviously difficult without a treadmill.

ASSESSMENT OF RESPIRATORY MUSCLE STRENGTH

A simple measure of respiratory muscle strength can be gauged by using a hand-held device to estimate maximal inspiratory and expiratory pressures. More complex measures requiring sophisticated equipment are discussed in Chapter 4c.

ASSESSMENT OF OXYGEN DELIVERY

Some patients with COPD may not demonstrate a resting hypoxaemia (<90%) but may desaturate on exercise. After exercise the oxygen saturation should not have dropped significantly; the frequently quoted value is less than 85%. If this occurs the patient should be considered a candidate for supplemental oxygen. The exercise test should be repeated with supplemental oxygen with measures of dyspnoea, exercise tolerance and desaturation monitored carefully to confirm that the portable oxygen cylinder has corrected the fall in saturation. Ambulatory oxygen cylinders in a carrying case are available for such occasions. The oxygen can be regulated at 1, 2 or 4 l/min and lasts for 4, 2 or 0.5 h respectively. If the fall in saturation is not corrected by the additional oxygen, careful consideration must be given to this candidate. The decision to prescribe an exercise regime for the patient must be taken in conjunction with the referring doctor, or the consultant medically responsible for the service. The isolated use of oxygen during the exercise component of rehabilitation does not necessitate or justify the use of continuous oxygen therapy at home.

Assessment of quality of life

The term quality of life has been described by the World Health Organization as 'an individual's perception of their position in life in the context of the culture and the value system in which they live and in relation to their goals, expectations, standards and concerns. It has a broad ranging concept affected in a complex way by a person's physical

Patient selection and
assessment for pulmonary
rehabilitation

health, psychological state, level of independence, social relationships, and their relationship to salient features of their environment' (World Health Organization, QOL Group, 1993). The quality of an individual's life is quite obviously multifactoral and quality of life research spans the whole spectrum; however, reports suggest that health is the most valued state (Kaplan *et al.*, 1993). This has been mirrored by purchasers of health care attaching increasing importance to positive health gains. Health-related quality of life is an attempt to judge how the patient is affected both physically and psychologically by the respiratory disease. Questionnaires are frequently employed as the mode of investigation. These can indicate the impact of a patient's breathlessness and other manifestations of respiratory disorders on daily life. Questionnaires were developed to aid the overall evaluation of patients' psychological, emotional and functional status and to reveal any hidden links between directly measured pathophysiological parameters and a patient's quality of life.

The first quality of life measure designed for the specific assessment of patients with chronic respiratory disorders was the Chronic Respiratory Disease Questionnaire (CRDQ; Guyatt *et al.*, 1987). This questionnaire consists of 19 questions and examines four aspects of patients' lives: dyspnoea, fatigue, emotion and mastery. Dyspnoea is evaluated by asking patients to identify the five most important activities which they do frequently and which are limited by dyspnoea. These can be volunteered independently or taken from a list. These activities are identified on the first administration and used when repeating the CRDQ. The responses for all the questions are based upon a seven-point Lickert scale. The questionnaire is both reproducible and responsive enough to detect changes in the quality of life. The questionnaire cannot be completed by the patient alone, and takes 25–30 min for the initial visit and 10–15 min for subsequent follow-ups.

The St George's Respiratory Questionnaire (SGRQ) assesses both COPD and asthma patients (Jones *et al.*, 1992). It is proposed that this test is more standardized than previous questionnaires; it consists of 76 items divided into three sections (symptoms, activity and impacts). The questionnaire, it is reported, correlates well with other reference values and also relates to more general measures of health, e.g. the Sickness Impact Profile (Bergner *et al.*, 1981).

The Breathing Problems Questionnaire (Hyland *et al.*, 1994) is, like the SGRQ, a self-completed questionnaire. It directs questions to the functional limitations and the emotional impact caused by the symptoms of chronic respiratory disease. It has 33 items and it is simple for the patient to complete in 10–15 min.

These three quality of life measures are described and reviewed in more detail in Chapter 3.

The failure of preselected patients to graduate through the pulmonary rehabilitation programme is a recurrent source of frustration to the health care team and demotivating to other participants on the course. Adherence is generally defined as 'the degree to which patient behaviour coincides with the clinical recommendations of the health care providers' (Rand, 1990). There is little evidence to suggest what is a good or appropriate level of adherence for pulmonary rehabilitation. Drop-out rates are not commonly reported, although a rate of around 33% has been informally suggested. Compliance is likely to be lower for patients with chronic disease, and even lower if the regimen is perceived as long and complicated. With this rate of attrition and limited resources, funds may be better utilized if those individuals likely to have difficulty adhering to the regimen can be identified.

Although patients with COPD benefit from a programme of exercise and education, motivation and compliance can be a problem, not least because of the absence of a critical incident, a common feature of patients recruited for cardiac rehabilitation. Patients frequently regard their situation as futile, particularly if they are severely disabled, thus their willingness to embark upon a course of rehabilitation is curtailed. Alternatively, if mildly affected, a low perception of severity and insufficient motivation are likely; they may believe that pulmonary rehabilitation is a waste of time. Kaplan and Simon (1990) suggested that non-compliance can be divided into three categories: patient-related, environment-related and patient–provider interaction-related. Patient-related factors embrace the patient's sex, age and race. Stone (1979) reported that no single variable could consistently predict compliance but it increased with age, socioeconomic status and education and was higher in a white than black population. The second factor proposes that the individual's environment influences compliant behaviour. The areas for consideration might be cultural, family or situational. Environmental cues may be related to individuals performing home exercise and incorporating this into their daily routine. Finally, it has been suggested that defects in the patient–provider relationship may provoke or discourage compliant behaviour. This can be in terms of the exchange of adequate knowledge and the success of the relationship, which may be particularly important for a series of treatment episodes over a short period of time.

The most widely practised measure is based upon the initial rapport developed between the patient and the health care professional. However, it has been repeatedly documented that physicians are wildly optimistic about patient compliance with medication (Mushlin and Appel, 1977); therefore 'gut reaction' to a patient is not enough to predict compliance. Patient characteristics have been examined to identify those non-compliant individuals, examining psychological, cognitive-motivational factors, somatic factors and behaviour itself (Dunbar, 1990). The literature does not appear to support the influence of personality traits as predictors but certain psychological states may influence compliance, particularly depression and anxiety. This was demonstrated by Blumenthal *et al.* (1982) in patients attending cardiac rehabilitation. More recently, Wolstenholme and Baines (1995) demonstrated similar findings for pulmonary rehabilitation.

Cognitive-motivational factors can also be potential predictors of patient compliance. The health belief model refined in 1984 by Janz and Becker suggests that individuals are more likely to exhibit compliant behaviour if they believe that they are susceptible to the illness; that the consequences of non-compliance are serious; that the treatment will reduce the risk or severity of the disease; and finally, if there is a net health benefit, i.e. if the benefits of compliant behaviour do not exceed the effort required to follow the treatment or advice. The influence of cognitive-motivational factors is complicated by the timing of individuals' evaluation of the health belief model; this model is perhaps most powerful around the time of diagnosis. Indeed, patients may be able successfully to predict their own compliance, particularly if they have some experience of the treatment regimen (Kaplan and Simon, 1990) and are aware of the benefits and consequences. Somatic factors as predictors of compliance run parallel to the perceived benefits and drawbacks; those patients who experience a reduction in symptoms are more likely to graduate from the programme, whilst those perceiving an increase in symptoms are more likely to drop out. This is of course complicated by individuals' perceptions of symptoms and their intensity. Alternatively, health behaviour can be used to predict subsequent adherence; previous compliance may be useful for the prediction of future compliance. Early compliant behaviour within rehabilitation will increase the probability of graduation.

WHAT CAN WE DO TO IMPROVE COMPLIANCE?

Improving compliance can generally be described in three categories: organizational, educational and behavioural intervention. Manipulating the organization to improve compliance focuses upon the convenience of the initial assessment, waiting times, times of the classes and some travel arrangements. Educational intervention is important for the transmission of knowledge, to improve patients' information concerning their own regimen. This begins before the patient attends for classes with adequate information conveyed by the referring doctor, which can be supported by a brief explanatory leaflet. Subsequent information, commonly disseminated during the educational component of the programme, can be consolidated by further leaflets, booklets and hand-outs, which can be collated into one file. Patients vary tremendously in the amount of information they bring to the programme and how much they wish to acquire. From our own experience we have been guilty of underestimating the depth of our patients' knowledge.

Specific and individualized information is necessary to strengthen compliance to an exercise training regimen and lifestyle adaptations. The regimen should be straightforward, thus augmenting its convenience and patient cooperation; this is further improved if the exercise sessions are supervised and continuously monitored. The final option is to employ behavioural strategies both to influence non-compliant behaviour and to maintain high compliance. One such study is reported by Atkins *et al.* (1984): five groups of COPD patients were identified and a walking regimen prescribed. The experimental groups were designed to improve compliance with the exercise regimen by using behavioural modification, cognitive-behavioural modification and cognitive modification. The control groups were attention control (attention but not designed to improve compliance) and a control group who were prescribed an exercise programme but advised to continue with this independently of hospital-based supervision. Compliance was observed to be greatest in the experimental groups compared to the controls and greatest in the cognitive-behavioural group (positive self-talk exercises, relaxation and contingency management). Although there are a variety of behavioural strategies, the most useful to pulmonary rehabilitation are likely to be tailoring, contracting, graduated regimen implementation, self-monitoring and reinforcement (Dunbar *et al.*, 1979).

Tailoring refers to the process of fitting the prescribed regimen and intervention strategies to specific patient characteristics (Dunbar *et al.*, 1979). This strategy is relatively underresearched and it is not clear which patients may benefit from this technique. Contracting or goal-setting requires the patient and provider to negotiate a treatment goal. This can be a volunteered goal or identified as part of a functional assessment or measure of quality of life. In this process both parties need to identify specific roles and a time limit for its achievement. Previous research suggests that specific challenging goals lead to a higher output (Locke, 1968) and greater learning (Kaplan and Rothkopf, 1974) than vague goals, such as 'do your best'. Theoretically, goal-setting can be summarized as a motivational mechanism, which as a concept can be used to describe the direction, amplitude and duration of an action (Locke *et al.*, 1981). In practice this strategy appears to offer a number of benefits: involving patients in decision-making for their own regimen, provoking a formal commitment to the programme, thus enhancing compliance and finally, a written document of behavioural expectations is produced to

Box 2.6

What we can do to improve compliance

Comprehensive and consistent explanation of the programme

Convenience of the classes (time, duration of session and the entire programme)

Travel arrangements

Provider's attitude to the patient

Prescription of a simple training programme (with supervision and self-monitoring)

Perception of the consequences (short- and long-term) of compliance outweighing the expected benefits

Enlisting family and social support

Other factors (including word of mouth, doctor's recommendation, etc.)

foster the feeling of self-control over the rehabilitation. A graduated implementation regimen, as expected, provides a negotiated platform for the sequential progression of the exercise regimen or lifestyle changes. Self-reporting allows patients to monitor their own progress; for example, in rehabilitation patients might record their home exercise programme. Until recently this method was used purely for data collection, although increasingly it is being seen as an adjunct to enhancing compliance. Reinforcement – any action that results in the desired behaviour being repeated – improves compliance.

Identify who needs extra individual treatment

The final consideration is directed towards the appropriate identification of those patients who would benefit from individual physiotherapy, occupational therapy, dietary advice, sex therapy or psychological support. In some areas the rehabilitation service may be organized so that the initial assessment is multidisciplinary. Alternatively, the assessment may be conducted by one person from the rehabilitation team. In this instance a simple mechanism must be in place, for example short questionnaire, to target those individuals correctly. To minimize the time of the initial assessment this questionnaire must be sensitive yet simple.

PHYSIOTHERAPY

Patients identified for individual physiotherapy treatment are commonly those patients who present with:

- Recurrent chest infections (several courses of antibiotics in the previous year).
- Difficulties with chest clearance.
- Inappropriate shortness of breath after exercise, commonly associated with a delayed recovery time.
- Abnormal breathing patterns.
- Inappropriate inhaler technique.
  (For further information see Chapter 6.)

DIETICIAN

The most common reasons for referral to the dietician in our experience are obesity or being underweight (BMI over 30 or below 20). An attempt should be made to filter those individuals that have experienced unexplained weight loss (more than 10%) or those that have altered their dietary habits and adopted a more liquid diet than before towards the dietician (for further information see Chapter 5).

OCCUPATIONAL THERAPY

The role of the OT is to 'assist individuals to achieve maximum independence in relevant activities of daily living following disability or illness'. As result of pulmonary rehabilitation an individual may be functionally more proficient. This should succinctly identify those individuals that have difficulties with the fundamental activities of daily living (for further information see Chapter 7).

SEX THERAPIST

Problems with sexual relationships are an underrecognized problem in this client group. Intimacy is important to us all but perhaps more so in patients with COPD to compensate for the social isolation and depression frequently associated with the disease. The acknowledgement of problems requires diplomatic and sensitive discussion and the suggestion that more specific help is available and valuable. Frequently the occupational therapy staff will offer a counselling service or alternatively a sex therapist/counsellor may be available.

PSYCHOLOGIST

A contribution from a psychologist is invaluable. Patients suffering from a chronic disease may exhibit signs of psychological distress, commonly depression and anxiety. Behavioural modifications may also be noted, most obviously a decline in social and leisure activities. Patients referred to the psychologist for individual counselling are likely to exhibit a significant emotional component to their disease that may well inhibit a successful outcome of any physical intervention.

*Patient selection and
assessment for pulmonary
rehabilitation*

Evaluation of the rehabilitation services

Continued evaluation of pulmonary rehabilitation is vital to the maintenance and progression of the service. Evaluation can be subdivided into:

■ Experimental (research-based).
■ Local (clinical service).
■ Audit.
■ Cost–benefit analysis.

This book is designed as a practical source of information and not a
guide to research and thus a full analysis of evaluation is beyond the
scope of this text. When providing a clinical service it is important to
evaluate the service in its entirety rather than focusing on the patients
who successfully graduate from the programme. One measure of success
is an improvement in outcome measures. Alternatively, one might argue
that it is important to assess the client group and their needs and evaluate whether or not the service is targeted appropriately. To do this, the
pattern of referral must be observed, along with factors such as the acceptance rate for the initial assessment and drop-out rate. If patients frequently do not attend for the initial assessment, questions such as: 'Is the
patient information leaflet adequate?', 'Is the timing of the class inappropriate?' and 'Are we targeting the right type of patient?' need answer-
ing. If the rate of attrition once the patients have started the course is
high, the structure of the programme needs to be re-evaluated. There is
very little point having a spectacularly successful service for a minority
of patients with COPD.

Audit of the programme embraces both an element of research and
aspects of local evaluation. The process of audit facilitates critical evaluation of the service, not only in terms of the immediate gains but also
the long-term benefits to the individual and the health service.

Cost–benefit analysis attempts to offset the cost of rehabilitation
against the demands for other health care resources. Pulmonary rehabilitation is in its infancy in the UK and these questions remain largely
unanswered. The experience in the USA suggests that there is a paral-
leled drop in bed-days as a result of graduating from a rehabilitation
programme.

Conclusion

The identification of those patients likely to benefit from rehabilitation
can be challenging and secured in part by a thorough assessment. We are
not very successful at eliminating, at the time of the initial assessment,

those individuals who are not committed to attend the programme regularly, to take responsibility for a home exercise programme or to take on board suggested changes in lifestyle. Unfortunately, these individuals cannot be identified by simple spirometry or exercise testing and require detailed interviewing. Until such a time that a specific test is available to assist with this dilemma, we will continue to recruit this category of patient. This small percentage of patients does not detract from the success of pulmonary rehabilitation. Careful selection and assessment can be profitably used to identify patient limitations and aspirations and improve the probability of pulmonary rehabilitation succeeding.

References

Altose, D.M. (1985) Assessment and management of breathlessness. *Chest* **88**:77s–83s.

Ambrosino, N., and Foglio, K. (1996) Selection criteria for pulmonary rehabilitation. *Respir. Med.* **90**:317–22.

American College of Sports Medicine. (1991) *Guidelines for Exercise Testing and Prescription*, 4th edn. Philadelphia: Lea & Febiger.

American Thoracic Society. (1987) Standards for the diagnosis and care of patients with chronic obstructive pulmonary disease (COPD) and asthma. *Am. Rev. Respir. Dis.* **136**:225–44.

Astrand, P.-O., and Rodahl, K. (1986) *Textbook of Work Physiology*, 3rd edn. New York: McGraw Hill.

Atkins, C.A., Kaplan, R.M., Timms, R.M., and Reinsch, S. (1984) Behavioral exercise programs in the management of chronic obstructive pulmonary disease. *J. Consult. Clin. Psychol.* **52**:591–603.

Bergner, M., Bobbitt, R.A., Carter, W.B., and Gilson, B.S. (1981) The sickness impact file: development and final revision of a health status measure. *Med. Care* **19**:787–806.

Blumenthal, J.A., Williams, R.S., Wallace, A.G. *et al.* (1982) Physiological and psychological variables predict compliance to prescribed exercise therapy in patients recovering from myocardial infarction. *Psychosom. Med.* **44**:519–27.

Borg, G.A.V. (1982) Psychophysical bases of perceived exertion. *Med. Sci. Sport Ex.* **14**:377–81.

Bruce, R.A., Kusumi, F., and Hosmer, D. (1973) Maximal oxygen intake and nomographic assessment of functional aerobic impairment in cardiovascular disease. *Am. Heart J.* **85**:546–62.

Butland, R.J.A., Pang, J., Gross, E.R. *et al.* (1982) Two-, six- and twelve- minute walking tests in respiratory disease. *Br. Med. J.* **284**: 1607–8.

Casaburi, R., Wasserman, K., Patessio, A. *et al.* (1989) A new perspective in pulmonary rehabilitation: anaerobic threshold as a discriminant in training. *Eur. Respir. J.* (suppl. 7):618–23s.

Casaburi, R., Patessio, A., Ioli, F. *et al.* (1991) Reduction in exercise lactic acidosis and ventilation as a result of exercise training in patients with chronic lung disease. *Am. Rev. Respir. Dis.* **143**:9–18.

Clark, C.J. (1991) Strategies for the evaluation of rehabilitation treatment. *Eur. Respir. Rev.* **1**(suppl. 6):475–81.

Cooper, J.D., Trulock, E.P., Triantafillou, A.N. *et al.* (1995) Bilateral pneumectomy (volume reduction) for chronic obstructive pulmonary disease. *J. Thorac. Cardiovasc. Surg.* **109**:106–19.

Davidson, A.C., Leach, R., George, R.J.D., Geddes, D.M. (1988) Supplemental oxygen and exercise ability in chronic obstructive airways disease. *Thorax* **43**:965–71.

Dunbar, J. (1990) Predictors of patient adherence: patient characteristics. In: *The Handbook of Health Behaviour Change* (eds S.A. Shumaker, E.B. Schron and J.K. Ockene). New York: Springer, pp. 348–60.

Dunbar, J., Marshall, G.D., and Hovell, M.F. (1979) Behavioral strategies for improving compliance. In: *Compliance in Health Care* (eds R.B. Haynes, D.W. Taylor, D.L. Sackett). Baltimore: Johns Hopkins University Press, pp. 174–86.

Flenley, D.C. (1990) *Respiratory Medicine*, 2nd edn. London: Baillière Tindall.

Foster, S., and Thomas, H.M. (1990) Pulmonary rehabilitation in lung disease other than chronic obstructive pulmonary disease. *Am. Rev. Respir. Dis.* **141**:601–4.

Guyatt, G.H., Berman, L.B., Townsend, M. *et al.* (1987) A measure of quality of life for clinical trials in chronic lung disease. *Thorax* **42**:773–778.

Howell, J.B.L. (1990) Breathlessness. In: *Respiratory Medicine* (eds R.A.L. Brewis, G.J. Gibson and D.M. Geddes). London: Baillière Tindall, pp. 221–8.

Hyland, M., Bott, J., Singh, S.J., and Kenyon, C.A.P. (1994) Development and validation of a patient-completed questionnaire for assessing quality of life in patients with chronic obstructive pulmonary diseas. *Qual. Life Res.* **3**:245–56.

Janz, N.K., and Becker, M.H. (1984) The health belief model a decade later. *Health Educ. Q.* **11**:1–47.

Jones, N.L. (1988) *Clinical Exercise Testing*, 3rd edn. Philadelphia: WB Saunders.

Jones, P.W., Quirk, F.H., Baveystock, C.M., and Littlejohns, P. (1992) A self completed measure of health status for chronic airflow limitation. The St Georges Respiratory Questionnaire. *Am. Rev. Respir. Dis.* **142**:1321–7.

Kaplan, R., and Rothkope, E.Z. (1974) Instructional objectives as directions of learners: effect of passage length and amount of objective relevant content. *J. Educ. Psychol.* **66**:448–56.

Kaplan, R.M., and Simon, H.J. (1990) Compliance in medical care: reconsideration of self predictions. *Ann. Behav. Med.* **12**:66–71.

Kaplan, R.M., Feeny, D., and Revicki, D.A. (1993) Methods for assessing relative importance in preference based outcome measures. *Qual. Life Res.* **2**:467–75.

Locke, E.A. (1968) Toward a theory of task motivation and incentives. *Organis. Behav. Human Perform.* **3**:157–89.

Locke, E.A., Shaw, K.N., Saari, L.M., and Latham, G.P. (1981) Goal setting and task performance: 1969–1980. *Psychol. Bull.* **90**:125–52.

McGavin, C.R., Gupta, S.P., and McHardy, G.J.R. (1976) Twelve-minute walking test for assessing disability in chronic bronchitis. *Br. Med. J.* **1**:822–3.

McGavin, C.R., Artvinli, M., Naoe, H., and McHardy, G.J.R. (1978) Dyspnoea, disability, and distance walked: comparison of estimates of exercise performance in respiratory disease. *Br. Med. J.* **2**:241–3.

Mahler, D.A., Weinberg, D.H., Wells, C.K., and Feinstein, A.R. (1984) The measurement of dyspnea: contents, interobserver agreement and physiological correlates of two new clinical indexes. *Chest* **85**:751–8.

Mathur, R.F., Revill, S.M., Vara, D.D. *et al.* (1995) Comparison of peak oxygen uptake during cycle and treadmill exercise in severe chronic obstructive pulmonary disease. *Thorax* **50**:829–833.

Medical Research Council. (1966) *Committee on Research into Chronic Bronchitis: Instructions for Use on the Questionnaire on Respiratory Symptoms.* Devon: W.J. Holman.

Mushlin, A.I., and Appel, F.A. (1977) Diagnosing potential noncompliance: physicians' ability in a behavioral dimension of medical care. *Arch. Intern. Med.* **137**:318–21.

Rand, C.S. (1990) Issues in the measurement of adherence. In: *The Handbook of Health Behaviour Change* (eds S.A. Shumaker, E.B. Schron and J.K. Ockene). New York: Springer, pp. 102–110.

Rochester, D.F. (1991) Effects of COPD on the respiratory muscles. In: *Chronic Obstructive Pulmonary Disease* (ed N.S. Cherniack). Philadelphia: WB Saunders, pp. 134–57.

Simpson, K., Killian, K., McCartney, N. *et al.* (1992) Randomised controlled trial of weight lifting in patients with chronic airflow limitation. *Thorax* **47**:70–75.

Sinclair, D.J.M., and Ingram, C.G. (1977) Controlled trial of supervised exercise training in chronic bronchitis. *Br. Med. J.* **i**:519–21.

Singh, S.J., Morgan, M.D.L., Scott, S.C. *et al.* (1992) The development of the shuttle walking test of disability in patients with chronic airways obstruction. *Thorax* **47**:1019–24.

Singh, S.J., Morgan, M.D.L., Hardman, A.E. *et al.* (1994) Comparison of oxygen uptake during a conventional treadmill test and the shuttle walking test in chronic airflow limitation. *Eur. Respir. J.* **7**:2016–20.

Snider, G.L., Faling, L.J., Rennord, S.I. (1994) Chronic bronchitis and emphysema. In: *Textbook of Respiratory Medicine*, vol. 2, 2nd edn, (eds J.F. Murray and J.A. Nadel). Philadelphia: WB Saunders, pp. 1331–97.

Stoller, J.K., Ferranti, R., and Feinstein A.R. (1986) Further specification and evaluation of a new clinical index for dyspnea. *Am. Rev. Respir. Dis.* **134**:1129–34.

Stone, G.C. (1979) Patient compliance and the role of the expert. *J. Soc. Issues* **35**:34–59.

Sweer, L., and Zwillich, C.W. (1990) Dyspnoea in the patient with chronic obstructive pulmonary disease etiology and management. *Clin. Chest Med.* **11**:363–74.

Swinburn, C.R., Wakefield, J.M., and Jones, P.W. (1984) Relationship between ventilation and breathlessness during exercise in chronic obstructive airways disease is not altered by prevention of hypoxaemia. *Clin. Sci.*

67:515–19.

Swinburn, C.R., Wakefield, J.M., and Jones, P.W. (1985) Performance, ventilation and oxygen consumption in three different types of exercise tests in patients with chronic obstructive lung disease. *Thorax* **40**:581–6.

The Toronto Lung Transplant Group. (1988) Experience with single lung transplantation for pulmonary fibrosis. *J.A.M.A.* **259**:2258–62.

Tydeman, D.E., Chandeler, A.R., Graveling, B.M. *et al.* (1984) An investigation into the effects of exercise training on patients with chronic airways obstruction. *Physiotherapy* **70**:261–64.

West, J.B. (1987) *Pulmonary Pathophysiology – The Essentials*, 3rd edn. Baltimore: Williams & Wilkins.

World Health Organization QOL GROUP. (1993) *Measuring Quality of Life: The Development of the World Health Organization Quality of Life Instrument (WHO QOL)*. Geneva: WHO.

Wijkstra, P.J., Ten Vergert, E.M., Van Altena, R. *et al.* (1995) Long term benefits of rehabilitation at home on quality of life and exercise tolerance in patients with chronic obstructive pulmonary disease. *Thorax* **50**:824–8.

Wolstenholme, R.J., Baines, S. (1995) Respiratory rehabilitation, psychological distress and compliance. *Eur. Respir. J.* **8**:355s.

3. Assessment of quality of life in chronic lung disease

M.E. Hyland

Department of
Psychology, University
of Plymouth, Devon

Practical Pulmonary Rehabilitation.
Edited by Mike Morgan and Sally Singh.
Published in 1997 by Chapman & Hall, London.
ISBN 0 412 61810 9.

The term quality of life (QOL) or, more specifically, health-related QOL, refers to the patient's subjective judgement of health status. QOL is an outcome measure that can be contrasted with physiological measures such as spirometry or the physician's judgement about the patient's well-being or functional capacity. QOL can be assessed in several ways. The simplest way is to interview patients and ask them questions about how their disease has affected their lives. In some clinical contexts, the use of interviews will provide invaluable insight, particularly if the interviewer has a good understanding of the kind of QOL deficits that occur in the particular disease under consideration, in this case chronic lung disease (a good review is provided by Williams, 1993). However, a known disadvantage of unstructured interviews is that the information gained often depends as much on the interviewer as on the patient. Consequently, more formal methods of assessment are needed to achieve reliability, and these more formal methods form the focus of this chapter.

The most common formal method of assessing QOL is through the use of a questionnaire. The use of QOL questionnaires for a variety of purposes reflects a long tradition going back some 20 years. There are two kinds of QOL questionnaire: generic questionnaires and disease-specific questionnaires. Historically, the first to be developed were generic questionnaires. Generic QOL questionnaires are designed for patients having any disease, and therefore may be used for patients with lung disease. A review of the several generic disease questionnaires that have been published may be found in Bowling (1995), and these include the Sickness Impact Profile or SIP (Bergner *et al.*, 1981), the Nottingham Health Profile or NHP (Hunt *et al.*, 1986) and MOS Short Form-36 or SF-36 (Ware and Sherbourne, 1992). One feature of generic questionnaires is that they will often include questions that are irrelevant to a particular specific disease, and they may omit topics that are relevant. By contrast, disease-specific questionnaires include only questions that are relevant to the particular disease and therefore tend to be more sensitive to change. Sensitivity to change is an important feature of instruments used to assess the efficacy of an intervention programme, and consequently there has been a substantial development of disease-specific instruments in recent years, including those that are suitable for patients with chronic lung disease. A summary of generic and disease-specific questionnaires is shown in Table 3.1, with a listing of the subscales of each of these questionnaires.

I begin this chapter by reviewing three disease-specific instruments for assessing QOL in patients with chronic lung disease: the structured interview procedure described in the Chronic Respiratory Disease Questionnaire or CDRQ (Guyatt *et al.*, 1987), the patient-completed St George's Respiratory Questionnaire or SGRQ (Jones *et al.*, 1992) and the patient-completed Breathing Problems Questionnaire or BPQ (Hyland *et*

*Assessment of quality of
life in chronic lung
disease*

Table 3.1 Summary of both generic and disease-specific questionnaires

		Subscales	
Instrument	*Authors*	*Domains*	*Constructs*
Generic			
Nottingham Health Profile (NHP)	Hunt *et al.* (1986)	*Part I* Physical mobility Pain Sleep Energy Social isolation Emotional reactions *Part II* Work Looking after the home Social life Home life Sex life Interests and hobbies Holidays	
MOS 36 Item Short-Form Health Survey (SF-36)	Ware and Sherbourne (1992)	Physical functioning Role functioning– physical Bodily pain General health Vitality Social functioning Role functioning– emotional Mental health	
Sickness Impact Profile (SIP)	Bergner *et al.* (1981)	Ambulation Mobility Body care Social interactions Communication Emotional behaviour Alertness behaviour Home management Recreation and pastimes Eating Sleep and rest Work	

		Subscales	
Instrument	Authors	Domains	Constructs

Table 3.1 *Continued*

Disease-specific

Instrument	Authors	Domains	Constructs
Breathing Problems Questionnaire (BPQ)	Hyland *et al.* (1994)	Walking Bending or reaching Washing and bathing Household chores Social interactions Effects of weather or temperature Effects of smells and fumes Effects of colds Sleeping Medicine Dysphoric states Eating Excretion urgency	Problems/ health knowledge Evaluations/ health appraisal
Chronic Respiratory Disease Questionnaire (CRDQ)	Guyatt *et al.* (1987)	Dyspnoea Emotional function Fatigue Mastery	
St George's Respiratory Questionnaire (SGRQ)	Jones *et al.* (1992)	Symptoms Activity Impact	

al., 1994). This chapter concludes with an account of problems to consider when using any of these assessments to evaluate the outcome of rehabilitation in patients with chronic lung disease.

The Chronic Respiratory Disease Questionnaire

The CRDQ (Guyatt *et al.*, 1987) was the first of the disease-specific QOL instruments to be published for chronic lung disease. Although in the form of a questionnaire, this instrument is in fact a structured interview and the questionnaire provides an account of how to ask questions and to score patients' responses. The items are grouped into four subscales: dyspnoea, emotional function, fatigue and mastery. The authors state that the questionnaire takes a maximum of 30 min, and usually 15–20 min, for the first administration, with subsequent administrations taking between 10 and 15 min, with a maximum of 20 min.

The first section provides the dyspnoea subscale. More specifically, this section measures dyspnoea when patients are carrying out activity. The patient is asked to identify activities that have caused breathlessness during the last 2 weeks. As a further probe, the patient is then presented with a list of activities that can cause breathlessness. The patient selects the five activities that are most important to him or her and then rates each of these five activities on a seven-point scale ranging from 1 = extremely short of breath to 7 = not at all short of breath.

In contrast to many other QOL questionnaires, the first section of the CRDQ is unusual in that the activities rated are selected by the patient. As a consequence, the patient rates only those activities that are important, rather than all activities, some of which may not be important to that particular patient. The subsequent 15 items of the CRDQ cover the content of the remaining three subscales (emotional function, fatigue and mastery) and are of the conventional Lickert-type item with a seven-point response format. For example, question 11 is an item from the emotional function subscale and asks: 'In general, how much of the time did you feel upset, worried or depressed during the last 2 weeks?' Responses can vary between 1 = all of the time to 7 = none of the time.

When administering the scale in a rehabilitation programme, patients are allowed to see their initial responses when they complete the questionnaire at the end of the programme. This procedure has advantages as well as drawbacks, and is not a recommended feature of the other two questionnaires. The advantage in seeing the previous response is that the earlier response acts as an anchor in making the later response, thereby reducing error and increasing sensitivity to change. The disadvantage is that this sensitivity to change may be spurious in that patients may express their gratitude for the time and attention of hospital staff by recording responses that show that some improvement has taken place. This potential confounding effect is less important in a double-blind clinical trial, but is a potential problem for rehabilitation, as rehabilitation cannot be carried out blind.

The St George's Respiratory Questionnaire

The SGRQ (Jones *et al.*, 1992) was designed for use by patients with chronic lung disease as well as those with asthma, and patients respond to 76 questions. The questions fall into three categories: respiratory symptoms, activities limited or caused by breathlessness, and emotional impacts of breathlessness.

The first eight questions assess symptoms: patients are asked about the experience of symptoms over the last year. Unlike the dyspnoea items of the CRDQ, the symptoms items of the SGRQ do not refer to activities. The symptoms assessed are cough, phlegm, wheeze and shortness of breath, and there are questions about frequency of attacks of chest trouble, all of which are rated on five-point scales.

The remaining questions assess activities and impacts. The activities questions ask for information about activities making the patient breathless as well as activity restriction. Examples of activity restriction include 'I take a long time to get washed or dressed' and 'My breathing makes it difficult to do things such as very heavy manual work, run, cycle, swim fast or play competitive sports'. The patient ticks any items that apply, so that he or she is in effect responding to each of these questions on a two-point (yes–no) scale.

The impacts questions ask for information about the emotional impact on the patient, such as 'my cough or breathing is embarrassing in public' and 'I get afraid or panic when I cannot get my breath'. The patient ticks any items that apply, so again the response format is two-point.

The Breathing Problems Questionnaire

The BPQ (Hyland *et al.*, 1994) was designed for patients with chronic lung disease and has 33 questions which are completed by the patient. The questions are of the incomplete sentence format; the first four are shown in Figure 3.1. The response format varies between a four-point scale and a six-point scale depending on the question.

The questions cover 13 domains: walking, bending or reaching, washing and bathing, household chores, social interactions, effects of weather and temperature, effects of smells and fumes, effects of colds, sleeping, medicine, dysphoric states, eating and excretion urgency. The authors also show that, in addition to classifying questions by domains, they can also be grouped on the basis of psychometric evidence into two constructs representing the physical problems of the disease and the emotional problems that are the consequence of the disease.

Comparisons between the disease-specific questionnaires

Each of the three questionnaires uses different styles of asking questions within the same questionnaire. In addition, the three questionnaires

1. Because of my breathing problems, I walk on the flat:

Please
tick one
only

- [ ] as fast as normal
- [ ] just below normal
- [ ] slowly
- [✓] very slowly

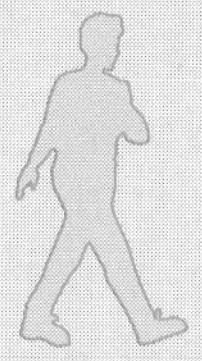

---

2. Because of my breathing problems, I walk on the flat without stopping for:

Please
tick one
only

- [ ] less than 20 paces (less than 10m)
- [ ] about 40 paces (about 20m)
- [ ] about 80 paces (about 40m)
- [✓] I never need to stop because of my breathing

---

3. When walking up a single flight of stairs (12 steps):

Please
tick one
only

- [ ] I can walk all the way up without getting breathless
- [ ] I can walk all the way up but am a bit breathless at the top
- [ ] I can walk all the way up but am really breathless at the top
- [ ] I need to stop once or twice on the way up
- [ ] I go up one step at a time
- [✓] Don't know/don't climb stairs

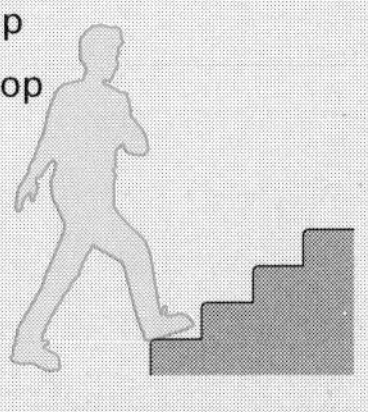

---

4. When I wash myself down I usually:

Please
tick one
only

- [ ] dry myself without any problems
- [ ] dry myself slowly
- [ ] sit and dry off
- [✓] need assistance to dry myself

Fig. 3.1 Selected items from the Breathing Problems Questionnaire.

differ from each other in terms of question style. The SGRQ uses a combination of four-point and two-point response formats, most having a two-point format; the BPQ uses a combination of four-point, five-point and six-point response formats; and the CRDQ uses a seven-point response format throughout, but with the special feature of patient-selected items for the five dyspnoea items. As a general rule, scales with more rather than fewer response options (up to a maximum of about seven) tend to be more sensitive to longitudinal change, and although this rule has not been confirmed with chronic lung patients, there are supportive comparative data in asthma (Juniper, in press). However, although longitudinal sensitivity is an advantage of the more complex response format, such formats take longer to complete and for some patients may be more difficult to understand. Thus, although the SGRQ has 76 items, the simple two-point response format for the majority of items means that the completion time for this scale is in the same order as the other scales which have less than half that number of questions. None of the authors give precise data relating to completion time which would permit comparison between the scales. However, as the authors of the CRDQ indicate, there are substantial differences between patients, some taking twice as long as others. In practice, a time allowance of 20 min should be adequate for most patients to complete any of the questionnaires. Although the CRDQ is the only instrument to be written specifically as a structured interview, the possibility of using a structured interview format exists with the other questionnaires: interviews tend to take longer than the equivalent material presented as a questionnaire.

All three questionnaires are content-valid instruments of QOL patients with chronic lung disease, so it is not surprising that there is considerable similarity in item content. Nevertheless, there are differences. All three questionnaires have items about symptoms, and all three have items about emotions, but there are differences in terms of the type of symptom or emotion sampled. For example, the BPQ has an item (item 24) about depression and the CRDQ has an item (item 11) about upset, worry or depression, but there is no depression item in the SGRQ. On the other hand, the SGRQ asks questions about cough, phlegm and frequency of attacks that are not asked by the other two questionnaires. A more important difference is that the CRDQ does not have any items relating to activity restriction. The occurrence of symptoms during activities is assessed by the CRDQ – as in the other two questionnaires – but not the degree of activity restriction.

Despite the similarity of many of the items, the three scales have substantially different subscales. The CRDQ has four; the SGRQ has three; and the BPQ has the option of 13 or two subscales. These differences arise in part because subscales are based either on researcher-generated

domains or patient-generated **constructs**. The CRDQ has domain subscales. The items have been grouped into four categories because the content of the items suggested those four categories to the authors. Similarly, the 13-domain subscales of the BPQ are based on the apparent content of the items as suggested to the authors. Domain classifications are arbitrary in that they depend on the judgement of authors who construct the scale. By contrast, construct classification relies on psychometric evidence obtained from patients' responses to the questionnaire and so construct classifications should be the same across questionnaires. The three subscales of the SGRQ are construct scales as the authors claim they obtained psychometric evidence for separating items into these three groups (Jones *et al.*, 1992). Similarly, the authors of the BPQ provide psychometric evidence for two constructs on the basis of patient responses to the BPQ (Hyland *et al.*, 1994). The difference between the three constructs of the SGRQ and the two constructs of the BPQ is readily explained. The SGRQ includes items which refer only to symptoms, and these items do not feature in the BPQ, where symptoms are only referred to in the context of activities. If this symptoms subscale is put to one side, then there is good correspondence between the psychometric findings of the SGRQ and the BPQ. The activities subscale of the SGRQ corresponds to the physical problems construct of the BPQ and the impacts subscale of the SGRQ corresponds to the emotional problems construct of the BPQ. In fact, psychometric evidence that QOL items separate into two groups, one reflecting physical problems and one reflecting emotional problems, is also a feature of generic QOL scales (McHorney *et al.*, 1993), so this finding does not appear to be specific to chronic lung disease, but rather a general finding about how patients judge their health status.

All three questionnaires are supported by validating evidence of one form or another, and so any could be used to assess outcome in rehabilitation. The absence of comparative data means that selection between the scales is largely a matter of preference, and it may be that different scales are preferred for different purposes. The best course of action for those wishing to assess QOL in chronic lung disease is to obtain copies of all three questionnaires and select the one whose style is most appropriate for the purpose for which it is to be used. Names and addresses of the authors of each of the three questionnaires are given at the end of this chapter.

QOL change and rehabilitation

One important conclusion to be drawn from the three questionnaires described above is that QOL is not a single entity. Each of the three ques-

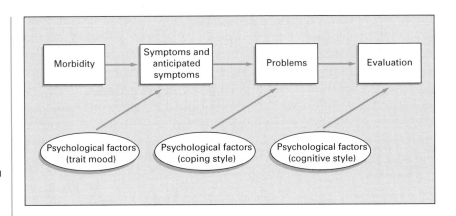

Fig. 3.2 Causal sequence of psychological constructs relevant to quality of life. From Hyland (1992), with permission.

tionnaires has subscales, and though the subscales are not identical, they can be related to each other. One of the most generalizable ways of thinking about subscales is in terms of the two constructs of physical problems and emotional problems. Indeed, although psychometric analysis was not used with the CRDQ, the emotional function, fatigue and mastery subscales all appear to reflect an emotional problem construct, and the dyspnoea subscale appears to be a physical problem construct, because the dyspnoea questions are asked in relation to activities.

Many physicians have the objective of improving the QOL of their patients. However, this aim is imprecise in that it leaves open the question of the different possible ways in which QOL is improved. A useful conceptual model for representing different ways in which QOL can change is shown in Figure 3.2 (Hyland, 1992). Figure 3.2 represents QOL as a causal sequence where physiological morbidity causes symptoms which cause physical problems which then cause emotional reactions. In addition, Figure 3.2 shows that QOL is a biopsychosocial interaction and that psychological factors interact during the causal sequence.

Consistent with the model shown in Figure 3.2, research in asthma shows that physiological improvement has a much greater impact on physical problems than on emotional problems (because physical problems are closer to morbidity in the causal sequence), but that emotional problems can be manipulated by some form of psychological intervention. For example, in a clinical trial, placebo conditions often lead to an improvement in emotional problems, probably because patients in clinical trials receive more emotional support from health professionals. However, when compared with the placebo condition, the active drug treatment improves only physical problems (Hyland, 1994). Thus, the effects of treatment on the constructs of QOL depend on the extent to which the treatment improves the physiological or psychological functioning of the patient.

Pulmonary rehabilitation has an effect on both physiological and psychological functioning. Even in programmes that are designed with purely physical goals in mind, the patient interacts with health professionals who are likely to be sympathetic, emotionally supportive and motivating. Pulmonary rehabilitation programmes are likely to be successful because of some combination of physical and psychological treatment of the patient where the psychological and physical aspects of rehabilitation interact. A patient is more likely to comply with advice about exercise if he or she has formed a good relationship with the health professional.

Any evaluation of pulmonary rehabilitation on QOL needs to consider QOL as a multicomponent concept where different aspects of rehabilitation may affect the different factors differently. The independence of the different components of QOL can be illustrated with the BPQ, where the physical problems subscale correlated 0.6 with a measure of exercise tolerance, the shuttle walking test, whereas the emotional problems subscale correlated only 0.2 with the shuttle walking test (Hyland *et al.*, 1994). However, the physical problems subscale did not correlate with the personality dimension of neuroticism, whereas the emotional problems subscale correlated 0.4 with neuroticism. Physical and emotional problems have different causes.

Improving QOL: some potential problems

In order to investigate the relative contributions of physical and psychological components of pulmonary rehabilitation, Ries *et al.* (1995) measured physiological and psychological outcomes when comparing an 8-week comprehensive rehabilitation programme with an 8-week educational programme. In the comprehensive programme patients received exercise training and physical and respiratory care instruction, whereas in the educational programme patients received only educational information. The results showed that patients attending the comprehensive programme had greater improvement on exercise performance and symptoms but not on QOL as measured by a generic scale of QOL. These results illustrate a finding which is common not only in pulmonary disease but also in other disease areas: in clinical studies it is often easier to obtain positive results on physical parameters rather than on QOL measures. Why should this be so?

One possible reason is that the patient's QOL reflects a pattern of behaviour that has been learned and has become well established over a period of time. If a patient has improved in terms of exercise capacity, this may be insufficient to cause a change in that established behaviour. Thus, the patient may improve exercise performance in the clinic, but this improvement then fails to generalize to the patient's life outside the clinic. Figure 3.1 shows that QOL is best viewed from the perspective of a biopsychosocial interaction rather than from the perspective of a purely biological model of medicine. Improvement to the biological condition of the patient may be a necessary but not a sufficient condition to reducing the patient's physical problems as experienced on a day-to-day basis. Moreover, improvement to the biological condition may have little impact on the patient's emotional problems, which may have causes other than that of physical condition.

The conclusion is that interventions and outcomes need to be **linked**. An intervention that focuses only on exercise performance may cause improvement only to clinic-assessed exercise performance. However, if the aim is to improve QOL, then for a positive effect to be obtained on a QOL outcome, the relationship between improved exercise performance and QOL change must be established for the particular patient. That is, health professionals should not assume that physical gains automatically translate into QOL gains. If QOL is an important outcome, rehabilitation programmes should contain a component that helps the patient translate physical gains into QOL gains.

Contacts for questionnaires

Chronic Respiratory Disease Questionnaire
Gordon Guyatt
Department of Clinical Epidemiology and Biostatistics
McMaster University Medical Centre
1200 Main Street West
Hamilton
Ontario
Canada L8N 3Z5

St George's Respiratory Questionnaire
Paul W. Jones
Division of Physiological Medicine
St George's Hospital Medical School
Cranmer Terrace
London SW17 0RE

Breathing Problems Questionnaire
Michael E. Hyland
Department of Psychology
University of Plymouth
Plymouth PL4 8AA

References

Bergner, M., Bobbit, R.A., Carter, W.B., and Gilson, B.S. (1981) The Sickness Impact Profile: development and final revision of a health status measure. *Med. Care* **19**:787–805.

Bowling, A. (1995) *Measuring Disease*. Milton Keynes, UK: Open University Press.

Guyatt, G.H., Berman, L.B., Townsend, M. *et al.* (1987) A measure of quality of life for clinical trials in chronic lung disease. *Thorax* **42**:773–8.

Hunt, S.M., McEwen, J., and McKenna, S. (1986) *Measuring Health Status*. London: Croom Helm.

Hyland, M.E. (1992) A reformulation of quality of life for medical science. *Qual. Life Res.* **1**:267–72.

Hyland, M.E. (1994) Antiasthma drugs: quality of life rating scales and sensitivity to longitudinal change. *PharmacoEconomics* **6**:324–9.

Hyland, M.E., Bott, J., Singh, S., Kenyon, C.A.P. (1994) Domains, constructs, and the development of the breathing problems questionnaire. *Qual. Life Res.* **3**:245–56.

Jones, P.W., Quirk, F.H., Baveystock, C.M., and Littlejohns, P. (1992) A self-complete measure for chronic airflow limitation – the St George's Respiratory Questionnaire. *Am. Rev. Respir. Dis.* **145**:1321–7.

Juniper, E.F. (in press) Quality-of-life considerations in the treatment of asthma. *PharmacoEconomics*.

McHorney, C.A., Ware, J.E., and Raczek, A.E. (1993) The MOS 36 item Short-Form Health Survey (SF-36). 2. Psychometric and clinical tests of validity in measuring physical and mental health constructs. *Clin. Care* **31**:247–63.

Ries A.L., Kaplan, R.M., Limberg, T.M.K., and Prewitt, L.M. (1995) Effects of pulmonary rehabiliation on physiological and psychological outcomes in patients with chronic obstructive pulmonary disease. *Ann. Intern. Med.* **122**:823–32.

Ware, J.E., and Sherbourne, C.D. (1992) The MOS 36-item Short-Form Health Survey (SF-36). *Med. Care* **30**:473–83.

Williams, S.J. (1993) *Chronic Respiratory Illness*. New York: Routledge.

4. Exercise training

4a. Theoretical rationale for training

A.E. Hardman

Department of Physical Education, Sports Science and Recreation Management, Loughborough University

Practical Pulmonary Rehabilitation.
Edited by Mike Morgan and Sally Singh.
Published in 1997 by Chapman & Hall, London.
ISBN 0 412 61810 9.

Introduction

The rationale for rehabilitative exercise is often predicated on the improvements in exercise performance and ability to cope with activities of daily living which are evident after training programmes. At minimal levels exercise helps avoid the debilitating spiral of incapacity, inactivity and aggravated disability which results from inactivity. When regular, frequent and sufficient in intensity it improves both functional capacity (peak performance) and endurance (stamina).

Even in the absence of a traditional training response, however, patients may benefit from increasing their physical activity levels; each bout of exercise stimulates favourable short-term metabolic and cardiovascular effects and repeated bouts may result in desensitization to the increased dyspnoea of exercise. Improvements in energy balance probably arise from improved matching of food intake to energy expenditure and there is the increased nutrient intake inevitably associated with greater energy turnover. Not least, improved confidence and self-esteem are valuable consequences of exercise rehabilitation. The purpose of this section is to review the functional and metabolic rationale for rehabilitative exercise in patients with chronic lung disease; issues related to nutrition and quality of life are addressed elsewhere.

Some definition of terms may be helpful; exercise performance is an absolute measure, for example, time needed to complete a given distance as quickly as possible. It reflects both habitual physical activity levels, i.e. fitness (the nurture factor) and genetic predisposition (the nature factor) as well as any restrictions imposed by pathophysiology. Endurance is the term reserved for the ability to sustain exercise which demands a high proportion of personal functional capacity (maximal oxygen uptake, $\dot{V}O_{2max}$) and a characteristic conferred by regular exercise, i.e. training.

Avoidance of deconditioning

This is surely the primary physiological goal of exercise rehabilitation for patients with chronic obstructive pulmonary disease (COPD), whose levels of physical activity are necessarily compromised by their disease. The consequences of inactivity are legion (Saltin and Rowell, 1980); muscle mass is reduced because the cross-sectional area of individual muscle fibres, and therefore of the the whole muscle, decreases. The effect is rapid and local; for example, 4–6 weeks of immobilization after knee surgery results in a decline of more than a quarter in the cross-sectional area of skeletal muscle fibres in the vastus lateralis muscle of

> ## Definitions
>
> Performance – time to complete given distance; maximum work
> rate achieved
> Endurance capacity – ability to sustain a high proportion of one's
> maximal oxygen uptake

Box 4a.1

the immobilized leg, with a corresponding decrease in total muscle cross-sectional area (Halkjaer-Kristensen *et al.*, 1980). The latter relates strongly to the muscle's capacity to develop tension, and therefore its strength, so that inactivity inevitably leads to impairment of strength.

Inactivity not only decreases muscle mass and strength but also impairs its metabolic quality. Studies of de-training show a marked decrease in muscle respiratory capacity as measured by the activity of enzymes of the citric acid cycle and the electron transport chain (Henriksson and Reitman, 1977). This is true for sedentary and well-trained subjects alike. In healthy, sedentary people, activities of the oxidative enzymes are higher in leg than in arm muscles, presumably because the muscles of the legs are used more in endurance activity than those of the arms. The importance of the respiratory capacity of muscle is that it appears to determine endurance; this has been shown most strikingly in animal studies where high correlations are evident between *in vitro* measures of respiratory capacity and running time to exhaustion. Contractile protein synthesis and the activity of enzymes of energy metabolism are both dependent on activity.

Whole-body inactivity, as in bed rest, results in marked decreases in functional capacity; classic studies in the late 1960s showed a drop in $\dot{V}O_{2max}$ of 27% after 3 weeks of bed rest (Saltin *et al.*, 1968), but even cessation of training whilst maintaining the normal activities of daily living results in a measurable decrease after 4–6 weeks (Henriksson and Reitman, 1977).

Functional loss associated with inactivity is not restricted to skeletal muscle. Mechanical loading is, arguably, the most important determinant of bone architecture and essential for maintenance of skeletal integrity (Lanyon, 1996). Physical inactivity results in a loss of calcium from bone, as has been demonstrated in humans by studies of astronauts during space flight and of patients subjected to bed rest. Loss is evident only in unloaded bone, showing that this strain-related effect is mediated locally. It is unlikely, however, that levels of physical activity attainable by patients with COPD, mild or severe, will be sufficient to increase bone density; a realistic goal is to slow down the age- and inactivity-related rate of loss.

Physical inactivity results in a rapid loss of:

Muscle mass and strength

Muscle respiratory capacity and therefore whole-body endurance

Maximal oxygen uptake

Bone mineral density

In the typical elderly patient with COPD inactivity-related decreases in functional capacities – of muscle groups or the whole body – are critically important. Although their decrease is gradual, because of disease progression and the natural decline due to ageing, when they fall below thresholds needed for tasks such as crossing a road safely, climbing stairs or rising from a low armless chair or toilet, there are sudden and deleterious consequences for the quality of life. Conversely, even small increases in capacities arising from rehabilitative exercise can take an individual just over such a threshold, with corresponding improvements in his or her capacity for independent living.

Functional capacity and endurance

Even low levels of exercise such as walking provoke marked increases in the body's metabolic rate; walking at 2 mph or 0.9 m/s, for instance, increases energy expenditure to about $2^{1}/_{2}$ times the resting rate. Consequently exercise is associated with profound changes in whole-body oxygen uptake, in this example from about 0.25 l/min at rest to more than 0.5 l/min during slow walking. Close coupling between oxygen uptake and cardiorespiratory responses ensures the matching of oxygen provision to demand when exercise is submaximal.

The relationship between oxygen uptake and exercise intensity is more or less linear during submaximal exercise which increases progressively in intensity (Fig. 4a.1). Therefore the highest oxygen uptake that the individual can attain, the $\dot{V}O_{2max}$ or $\dot{V}O_{2peak}$, dictates the highest exercise intensity which each individual can attain. This quantity is an important reference point for other reasons; in healthy people the sundry physiological responses to a bout of exercise appear to be dictated by the proportion of $\dot{V}O_{2max}$ that it constitutes rather than by any absolute measure of its intensity, e.g. speed of running or walking, work rate on a cycle ergometer. This is also likely to be the case for patients with COPD, but there is no evidence.

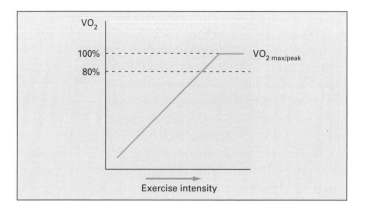

Fig. 4a.1 Schematic representation of oxygen uptake response to exercise of increasing intensity. $\dot{V}O_{2max/peak}$ limits the highest intensity achieved. Endurance capacity is the ability to sustain a high proportion, say 80% of $\dot{V}O_{2max/peak}$.

As mentioned above, the term endurance capacity describes the ability of individuals to sustain exercise which demands a high proportion of their $\dot{V}O_{2max}$ or $\dot{V}O_{2peak}$.

Limitations to maximal oxygen uptake

Investigation of the limitations to $\dot{V}O_{2max}$ are of interest in normal subjects and in patients alike because the understanding gained leads to effective strategies to push back these limits, for example by training or therapeutic intervention.

In normally active, healthy people, the limitation to oxygen uptake during exercise with the body's large muscles is probably the capacity of the cardiovascular system to deliver oxygen to exercising skeletal muscle (Saltin, 1990); when this is manipulated experimentally, for instance by breathing a gas mixture with 50% oxygen or by autologous blood reinfusion, $\dot{V}O_{2max}$ is increased significantly.

Training by already physically active men increases $\dot{V}O_{2max}$ by improving maximal cardiac output – rather than the maximal arteriovenous difference for oxygen, in support of this view. Muscle blood flow and oxygen uptake per unit mass of this tissue are both profoundly greater during exercise with the quadriceps muscles alone than during whole-body exercise (Andersen and Saltin, 1985), showing that muscle's metabolic capacity exceeds that which it is able to achieve during dynamic, aerobic exercise with the body's major muscle groups – say 25–30 kg muscle in a healthy young man.

When previously sedentary people become more active, however, increases in both maximal cardiac output and maximal arteriovenous difference for oxygen are evident, suggesting that the rate at which oxygen can be utilized in adenosine triphosphate (ATP) resynthesis may initially be a limiting factor in individuals whose habitual activity levels have been extremely low.

In patients with COPD pathophysiological changes mean that abnormalities of ventilatory mechanics, respiratory muscles, alveolar gas exchange and cardiac function are present to varying degrees (Belman, 1993). Theoretically, any of these could limit oxygen uptake capacity and their relative importance as potentially limiting factors probably differs from patient to patient. Among the most important are abnormal mechanics of ventilation, primarily attributable to expiratory airflow obstruction, but with important consequences for inspiratory muscle work as well as the obvious excessive use of expiratory musculature. Ventilation during maximal exercise reaches a high percentage of the maximum voluntary ventilation at rest, strongly suggesting a ventilatory limitation to oxygen transport. Consequently the term $\dot{V}O_{2peak}$ may be preferred to $\dot{V}O_{2max}$ for this group.

During submaximal exercise impaired gas exchange due to a reduced alveolar ventilation means a greater than normal increase in total minute ventilation to maintain carbon dioxide output as exercise intensity increases. Heart rates for a given $\dot{V}O_2$ are higher, possibly because of the characteristic increase in vascular resistance in COPD.

There are obvious reasons for the emphasis on impaired ventilatory mechanics and the associated dyspnoea but high intensity of leg muscle effort, and presumably leg fatigue, has been shown to be a reason why patients with COPD were unable to continue with an incremental exercise test on a cycle ergometer (Killian *et al.*, 1992). Leg fatigue was less commonly reported as a reason for stopping exercise in patients with severe COPD than in patients with mild or moderate airflow limitation but it was limiting in 11 of 31 patients with severe disease. This observation is not surprising in the light of the effects on muscle respiratory capacity of the inactivity which accompanies chronic disorders.

Limitations to endurance

Endurance during prolonged (≥ 1.5 h) exercise at about 70% of $\dot{V}O_{2max}$ is limited in normal subjects by substrate availability, in particular by muscle glycogen concentration. When this is manipulated by dietary change, parallel changes in endurance are observed (Åstrand and Rodahl, 1986); compared with a normal diet, 3 days on a low-carbohydrate (high-fat and protein) diet curtails endurance time during cycling exercise (compared with a normal mixed diet); if the low-carbohydrate diet is then followed by 3 days on a high-carbohydrate diet, endurance is vastly improved. Thus, fatigue in prolonged high-intensity exercise is associated with muscle glycogen depletion, either in the muscle as a whole or selec-

Limitations to oxygen uptake capacity

Healthy people – usually maximal cardiac output
In chronic obstructive pulmonary disease – abnormal mechanics
of ventilation; local muscle fatigue (more likely in patients with
mild/moderate airflow limitation)

Box 4a.3

tively in particular types of fibres. Despite the availability of vast amounts of energy substrate as blood-borne fatty acids, endogenous carbohydrate appears to be the preferred substrate of skeletal muscle when the rate of ATP resynthesis is high. When this is not available, the individual will slow down or, in a laboratory constant-speed or constant-work-rate test, stop altogether.

During sustained exercise of even higher intensity, say $\geq 80\%$ $\dot{V}O_{2max}$, fatigue is more likely attributable, either directly or indirectly, to the acidosis arising from high glycolytic rates in the exercising muscle than to substrate depletion. Lactic acid, the end-product of glycolysis, is completely dissociated at physiological pH and so protons and lactate anions are formed at the same rate. Thus the pH in exercising muscle falls – to levels suggesting that the activities of rate-limiting enzymes such as glycogen phosphorylase and phosphofructokinase are reduced – creating a negative feedback which slows down the glycolytic rate; excitation–contraction coupling may also be impaired (the sarcoplasmic reticulum binds more calcium at low pH) and/or the contractile apparatus itself may be affected (protons compete with calcium ions for binding sites on the regulatory protein troponin, interfering with contraction). Secondary effects of this metabolic acidosis arise when the protons diffuse out of muscle; they are buffered in blood mainly by bicarbonate, increasing carbon dioxide production and so the ventilatory drive.

Both causes of fatigue – substrate depletion and the consequences of acidosis – are related to the oxidative capacity of muscle; oxidative degradation of 1 mol of glucose from glycogen results in a net yield of ATP of 37 mol ATP, compared with only 3 mol if the glucose is converted from pyruvate to lactate. Thus, the greater the rate of ATP resynthesis that can be sustained oxidatively, the less the need to complement this by increased glycolysis and the slower the rate of glycogen degradation at a standard work rate.

Data on endurance – as defined above, i.e. the capability to sustain exercise eliciting a high proportion of $\dot{V}O_{2peak}$ – in patients with COPD is limited. Many authors report endurance but to the author's knowledge only two have adopted a valid measure (Toshima *et al.*, 1990; Punzal *et al.*, 1991); in both studies endurance was determined as the time to volitional fatigue during treadmill walking at a speed selected in relation to each patient's performance on a preliminary incremental test to $\dot{V}O_{2peak}$. Other authors have used the term endurance to describe time to fatigue on an incremental test (e.g. Cox *et al.*, 1993) – properly an evaluation of peak performance. In COPD endurance is inevitably limited by the combination of restricted activity and pathophysiology so that patients cannot sustain exercise for long periods – certainly not long enough for substrate depletion to be a cause of fatigue. Likely limiting factors are peripheral muscle fatigue and/or dypsnoea.

Effects of endurance training – response in normals

In healthy people $\dot{V}O_{2max}$ can be increased with training by 6–30%, depending on the training regimen and the initial level of fitness. The most important adaptation appears to be an increase in maximal cardiac output which arises from increased maximal stroke volume; maximal heart rates are not changed. Endurance is improved by two mechanisms: first, a given bout of exercise constitutes a smaller percentage of the new, increased $\dot{V}O_{2max}$; this moderates the level of physiological stress provoked so that, for example, heart rate will be lower and plasma catecholamine concentrations less. (The oxygen cost of a given submaximal exercise is seldom altered, despite a reduced ventilation and therefore lower oxygen cost of breathing; this may be because decreases are too small to be detected or because they are hidden by increases in the oxygen consumption of skeletal muscle as oxidative capacity improves.) Second, local changes in the trained muscle profoundly enhance its oxidative capacity; activities of oxidative enzymes are increased, because of an increase in mitochondrial protein, and the microcirculation is improved. Both mean a greater capacity for oxidative ATP resynthesis with a correspondingly decreased reliance on glycolysis during standardized exercise.

Skeletal muscle's potential for change should be emphasized. It is profoundly adaptable; the $\dot{V}O_{2max}$ of athletes may be twice that of sedentary controls but the activity of mitochondrial enzymes is three- to fourfold higher. The stimulus appears to be a chronic demand for high oxygen consumption by the muscle; the resulting adaptation is therefore restricted to the muscles which are trained, as shown by studies where one leg is trained and not the other – enzyme activities remain unchanged in the untrained leg – and of athletes who train only specific muscle groups. Canoeists, for example, have mitochondrial enzyme activities in their leg muscles similar to those measured in sedentary people but activities in their arm muscles which are characteristically much higher.

In patients with COPD the presence of ventilatory impairment, increased pulmonary vascular resistance and possibility of hypoxaemia during even mild exercise suggests a very different scenario. These restrictions may mean that some, or even most, may not be able to exercise sufficiently to create the stimulus to muscle metabolism necessary to stimulate metabolic adaptations in skeletal muscle. Based on studies of exercise rehabilitation, however, it is clear that these patients **do** demonstrate a training effect – defined as improvements in the capability for exercise, rather than by any specific physiological or metabolic adaptations.

Over the last three decades there have been many studies of exercise training, although few have employed a control group. For detailed discussion of their findings the reader is referred to recent reviews (Ries, 1990; Carter *et al.*, 1992; Connors and Hilling, 1992; Whipp and Casaburi, 1994). A striking feature of the literature is that there is no measurable improvement in pulmonary function and gas exchange as a result of training; exercise does not influence the underlying pathology – and would not be expected to. On the other hand, improvements in the performance of exercise tests have been almost universally reported, although there is no agreement on the mechanisms responsible. This may be, in part, because a variety of protocols have been used; some authors have reported the stage which can be reached on an incremental exercise test (which measures peak performance, as mentioned above), others the time for which exercise of a constant intensity can be sustained (which measures endurance), yet others 12- or 6-min walking tests (which measure a combination of the two). This means that the causes of fatigue are not the same in all studies and consequently that training-induced adaptations which delay fatigue will also differ.

Probably the strongest evidence of a benefit from exercise training in COPD (Fig. 4a.2) comes from a randomized controlled study of 119 patients (Toshima *et al.*, 1990). The effects of a comprehensive rehabilitation programme including exercise were compared with a control programme involving only education. After 8 weeks patients in the rehabilitation group nearly doubled their endurance time during treadmill walking, compared with minimal increase in controls. Six months later, the treated group maintained this advantage, suggesting a lasting benefit, although this was not reflected in measures of quality of well-being. Improvements in endurance time could not be attributed to practice by the training group in treadmill walking.

Other studies which have compared changes in a rehabilitation group with those in a control group of patients also report improvement in exercise test performance with training (Cockcroft *et al.*, 1981; Cox *et al.*, 1993). The former investigators studied ex-coal workers with a mean age

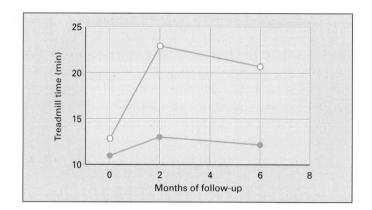

of 60, the treatment group spending 6 weeks in a rehabilitation centre where they undertook progressive exercise training – cycling, rowing, swimming and walking. On leaving the centre they were encouraged to continue with stair-climbing and walking at home. After 8 weeks. $\dot{V}O_{2peak}$ showed a small increase and 12-min walking distance a large increase. Cox and colleagues (1993) studied a mixed group of patients with asthma and mild COPD; the rehabilitation group improved significantly in $\dot{V}O_{2peak}$, maximal work rate and the work rate at which a blood lactate concentration of 4 mmol/l was reached. They also showed improvements in well-being, number of days worked and decreased consumption of medical care. These patients were, however, atypical; they were young (mean age just over 40), with only slight impairment of pulmonary function but with a history of high levels of days at home and in hospital because of dyspnoea. Moreover, they exercised for 4–5 h/day, doing team and individual sports, swimming, walking, cycling, skill and relaxation exercises – an exercise regimen neither feasible nor desirable for the typical patient with COPD.

Thus, controlled studies, together with more numerous uncontrolled studies, strongly suggest that exercise training both improves the level of exercise that can be achieved by patients with COPD and increases the time for which a given level of exercise can be sustained. A recent meta-analysis of 14 randomized controlled trials concluded that rehabilitation leads to improvements in functional exercise capacity which were greater than those associated with therapies such as bronchodilators or oral theophylline (Lacasse *et al.*, 1996).

Improvements may be attributable in part to an increased $\dot{V}O_{2peak}$ and/or because of a reduction in the oxygen cost of standard, submaximal exercise. The oxygen cost of exercise decreases both because of improvements in skill, i.e. increased efficiency, and because of a decrease in the oxygen requirement of respiratory muscles secondary to reduced ventilation. Overall, the effect is to reduce the proportion of $\dot{V}O_{2peak}$

elicited by a given bout of exercise, so that the individual is better able to sustain the exercise. Whether or not training by most patients can provoke metabolic changes in skeletal muscle is not known; few studies report changes in blood lactate concentrations (Casaburi *et al.*, 1991; Cox *et al.*, 1993) and they have employed rather rigorous training regimens in younger-than-average patients. Moreover, muscle biopsy study of oxidative enzyme concentrations in trained muscles revealed no significant improvements (Belman and Kendregan, 1981).

Theoretically, however, enforced inactivity in these patients must mean that the oxidative capacity of their skeletal muscles is poor, with correspondingly large potential for activity-related improvements. No pathophysiology of muscle metabolism is evident (Thompson *et al.*, 1993) and age *per se* does not appear to diminish the adaptive potential of this tissue. Respiratory muscles do not appear to be an important influence on the rise in blood lactate during exercise in patients with COPD (Engelen *et al.*, 1995), so that (deconditioned) exercising muscles are the likely source. In the light of the high prevalence of perception of leg effort as a limitation to exercise in patients with varying degrees of disease severity, local metabolic changes in trained muscle may therefore be an undervalued (and underresearched) aspect of adaptation.

Studies of the specificity of training lend support to this view. Upper-limb activity further hampers already impaired diaphragmatic function, yet repetitive arm movements are important in activities of daily living. Lake and colleagues (1990) therefore examined the effects of arm training alone with combined training of upper and lower limbs, comparing both with an untrained control group. Arm training improved upper-limb endurance but only the training regimen that included leg training improved walking distance. This is in line with classic studies of normal subjects which have shown that metabolic adaptations (the main determinants of endurance) are restricted to the trained muscles (Saltin *et al.*, 1976). In patients with COPD improved endurance for arm work has been reported to be accompanied by a decreased metabolic cost of standard arm exercise. Ventilatory muscle function, however, does not appear to improve, suggesting that improved endurance is either due to more skilled performance of the task or to metabolic adaptations similar to those described for normal subjects.

For normal subjects, there is considerable experience of exercise prescription, the intensity of exercise needed to elicit a training effect usually being defined in relation to $\dot{V}O_{2max}$. No consensus exists as to the optimal training regimen for patients with COPD. Different intensities of training have been examined, ranging from low, often self-selected, to high, sometimes defined as above an anaerobic threshold. As might be expected, more intense training results in more marked adaptive responses (Casaburi *et al.*, 1991). On the other hand, unstructured

Adaptations to endurance training

Healthy people	Increase in $\dot{V}O_{2max}$
	Increase in oxidative capacity of trained muscles, lower blood lactate response
	Improvements in both peak performance and endurance capacity
In chronic obstructive pulmonary disease	No change in pathophysiology
	No change in ventilatory muscle function
	Small increase in peak oxygen uptake
	Large improvement in endurance capacity
	Metabolic changes in skeletal muscle?

Box 4a.4

programmes where patients select their own exercise level are effective and clearly more practicable (Niederman *et al.*, 1991). They also minimize injury risk and avoid the discomfort of hard exercise which probably leads to poor compliance.

Most studies have looked at endurance training but there may be a role for strength training too. At least one study shows benefits in symptoms (as well as in cycle endurance) with arm- and leg-strengthening exercises (Simpson *et al.*, 1992). Strength training probably has a place in the rehabilitation programme, although exercise leaders need to bear in mind the cardiovascular sequelae of prolonged isometric contractions, particularly when these are performed with the arms.

Acute effects of each exercise bout

At the beginning of this chapter short-term acute effects of each exercise bout which may persist for some hours after exercise were referred to. These include decreased blood pressure during the post-exercise period; changes in insulin/glucose dynamics because of improved insulin sensitivity in the exercised muscle; and a decreased plasma triglyceride response to dietary fat. All these effects may be expected to be most clearly seen after sustained aerobic exercise has been performed with the body's major muscle groups (Haskell, 1994).

Implications for therapeutic exercise in COPD

What are the implications for the exercise component of pulmonary rehabilitation? First, benefits can be acquired from a whole range of dif-

---

Effects of each exercise bout (maximized if exercise is frequent)

Decrease in blood pressure

Improved glucose/insulin dynamics

Decreased postprandial plasma triglyceride response

Exercise prescription in chronic obstructive pulmonary disease

Individualized, but laboratory assessment not normally a prerequisite

Dynamic endurance exercise with large muscle groups, typically walking, but preferably also including arms

Exercises to increase strength – low resistance, emphasis on number of repetitions

Maintain generally more active lifestyle

---

ferent approaches (Table 4a.1); laboratory assessment is not a prerequisite and the prescription of the intensity of exercise – frequently the aspect which gives rise to most concern – does not demand a 'two-decimal-point' level of precision. One useful approach may be based on dyspnoea ratings (Horowitz *et al.*, 1996). There are good reasons for recommending whole-body endurance exercise with the body's large muscles: this ensures a sustained increase in cardiac output with little increase in blood pressure, brings about a worthwhile expenditure of energy and maximizes any acute effects which derive from exercise-induced changes in the exercised muscle (e.g. increases in insulin sensitivity, decreases in the rise in plasma triglyceride after a meal). There should be room for specific arm training in view of the importance of upper-body movements in the activities of everyday living. Exercises to increase strength are worthwhile but the emphasis should be on many repetitions against low resistance.

Finally, the overriding concern is that patients should increase their physical activity levels and then maintain, within the limits of their disease, a generally more active life. Older (>75 years) patients benefit at least as much as younger ones (Couser *et al.*, 1995). It is highly desirable that prescription be on an individual basis – to accommodate interindi-

Table 4a.1 Exercise training in chronic obstructive pulmonary disease			
	Casaburi et al. (1991)	Punzal et al. (1991)	Niederman et al. (1991)
No. of patients	9	57	33
FEV_1/FVC	58%	44%	50%
Intensity	High (60% of difference between anaerobic threshold and $\dot{V}O_{2peak}$)	High (mean of 85% of maximal work load in METs)	Initially ≤50% maximum work rate in cycle ergometry, regulated by RPE, increased when 20 min reached
Frequency and duration	45 min/day, 5 times a week for 8 weeks	Daily (duration not specified) for 8 weeks	≤20 min on each of three modes, 3 times a week, for 9 weeks
Mode of training	Cycle ergometer	Treadmill plus free walking	Cycle ergometer, treadmill, arm ergometer/free weights
Test	Incremental cycle ergometer 6.6–11.4-min increase Anaerobic threshold increased	Treadmill endurance at anaerobic threshold or maximum treadmill load 12.1–22.0-min increase	Incremental cycle ergometer and 12-min walk 5.0–12.4-min increase cycle time 1350–1700-m increase walk distance
$\dot{V}O_{2peak}$	10% increase	10% increase	19% increase ($P > 0.1$)

FEV_1 = Forced expiratory volume in 1 s; FVC = forced vital capacity; $\dot{V}O_{2peak}$ = peak oxygen consumption; METs = multiples of resting metabolic rate – assumed to be 3.5 ml/kg per min (American College of Sports Medicine, 1995); RPE = rating of perceived exertion (Borg, 1982). Modified from Belman (1993).

vidual differences in functional capacity, pathophysiology and lifestyle. Varying the type of activity may help with motivation and also decrease injury risk. High-intensity exercise may be maximally effective in improving functional capacities but it will usually be inappropriate and poorly adhered to. For the majority of patients, frequent (and regular) short bouts of low/moderate exercise may be expected to produce a cumulative, good enough degree of functional improvement to confer worthwhile benefit.

References

American College of Sports Medicine. (1995) *Guidelines for Exercise Testing and Prescription*, 5th edn. Baltimore: Williams & Wilkins.

Andersen, P., and Saltin, B. (1985) Maximal perfusion of skeletal muscle in man. *J. Physiol.* **366**:233–49.

Åstrand, P-O., and Rodahl, K. (1986) *Textbook of Work Physiology*, 3rd edn. New York: McGraw-Hill, pp. 183–5, 543–56.

Belman, M.J. (1993) Exercise in patients with chronic obstructive pulmonary disease. *Thorax* **48**:936–46.

Belman, M.J., and Kendregan, B.A. (1981) Exercise training fails to increase skeletal muscle enzymes in patients with chronic obstructive pulmonary disease. *Am. Rev. Respir. Dis.* **123**:256–61.

Borg, G.A. (1982) Psychophysical bases of perceived exertion. *Med. Sci. Sports Ex.* **14**:377–81.

Carter, R, Coast, J.R., and Idell, S. (1992) Exercise training in patients with chronic obstructive pulmonary disease. *Med. Sci. Sports Ex.* **24**:281–91.

Casaburi, R., Patessio, A., Ioli, F. *et al.* (1991) Reductions in lactic acidosis and ventilation as a result of exercise training in patients with obstructive lung disease. *Am. Rev. Respir. Dis.* **143**:9–18.

Cockcroft, A.E., Saunders, M.J., and Berry, G. (1981) Randomised controlled trial of rehabilitation in chronic respiratory disability. *Thorax* **36**:200–3.

Connors, G., and Hilling, L. (1992) *Guidelines for Pulmonary Rehabilitation. Programs.* Champaign, Illinois: Human Kinetics.

Couser, J.I., Guthmann, R., Hamadeh, M.A., and Kane, C.S. (1995) Pulmonary rehabilitation improves exercise capacity in older elderly patients with COPD. *Chest* **107**:730–34.

Cox, N.J.M., Hendricks, J.C. Binkhorst, R.A. and van Herwaarden, C.L.A. (1993) A pulmonary rehabilitation program for patients with asthma and mild chronic obstructive pulmonary diseases (COPD). *Lung* **171**:235–44.

Engelen, P.K.J., Casaburi, R., Rucker, R., and Carithers, E. (1995) Contribution of the respiratory muscles to the lactic acidosis of heavy exercise in COPD. *Chest* **108**:1246–51.

Halkjaer-Kristensen, J., Ingemann-Hansen, T., and Saltin, B. (1980) Cross-sectional and fibre size changes in the quadriceps muscle of man with immobilization and physical training. *Muscle Nerve* **3**:275.

Haskell, W.L. (1994) Health consequences of physical activity: understanding and challenges regarding dose-response. *Med. Sci. Sports Ex.* **26**:649–60.

Henriksson, J., and Reitman, J.S. (1977) Time course of changes in skeletal muscle succinate dehydrogenase and cytochrome oxidase activities and maximal oxygen uptake with physical activity and inactivity. *Acta Physiol. Scand.* **99**:91–7.

Horowitz, M.B., Littenberg, B., and Mahler, D.A. (1996) Dyspnea ratings for prescribing exercise intensity in patients with COPD. *Chest* **109**:1169–75.

Killian, K.J., Leblanc, P., Martin, D.H. *et al.* (1992) Exercise capacity and ventilatory, circulatory, and symptom limitation in patients with chronic airflow limitation. *Am. Rev. Respir. Dis.* **146**:935–40.

Lacasse, Y., Wong, E., Guyatt, G.H. *et al.* (1996) Meta-analysis of respiratory rehabilitation in chronic obstructive pulmonary disease. *Lancet* **348**:1115–19.

Lake, F.R., Henderson, K., Briffa, T. *et al.* (1990) Upper-limb and lower-limb exercise training in patients with chronic airflow obstruction. *Chest* **97**:1077–82.

Lanyon, L.E. (1996) Using functional loading to influence bone mass and architecture: objectives, mechanisms and relationship with estrogen of the mechanically adaptive process in bone. *Bone* **18**:375–435.

Niederman, M.S., Clemente, P.H., Fein, A.M. *et al.* (1991) Benefits of a multi-disciplinary pulmonary rehabilitation program. Improvements are independent of lung function. *Chest* **99**:798–804.

Punzal, P.A., Ries, A.L., Kaplan, R.M., and Prewitt, L.M. (1991) Maximum intensity exercise training in patients with chronic obstructive pulmonary disease. *Chest* **100**:618–23.

Ries, A.L. (1990) Position paper of the American Association of Cardiovascular and Pulmonary Rehabilitation. Scientific basis of pulmonary rehabilitation. *J. Cardiopulmon. Rehab.* **10**:418–41.

Saltin, B. (1990) Cardiovascular and pulmonary adaptation to physical activity. In: *Exercise, Fitness and Health* (eds C. Bouchard, R.J. Shephard, T. Stephens, J.R. Sutton and B.D. McPherson). Champaign, Illinois: Human Kinetics, pp. 187–203.

Saltin, B., and Rowell, L.B. (1980) Functional adaptations to physical activity and inactivity. *Fed. Proc.* **39**:1506–13.

Saltin, B., Blomqvist, G., Mitchell, J.H. *et al.* (1968) Response to exercise after bed rest and after training. *Circ. Res.* **38** (suppl. 7):1–78.

Saltin, B., Nazar, K., Costill, D.L. *et al.* (1976) The nature of the training response: peripheral and central adaptations to one-legged exercise. *Acta Physiol. Scand.* **96**:289–305.

Simpson, K., Killian, K., McCartney, N. *et al.* (1992) Randomised controlled trial of weightlifting exercise in patients with chronic airflow limitation. *Thorax* **47**:70–5.

Thompson, C.H., Davies, R.J.O., Kemp, G.J. *et al.* (1993) Skeletal muscle metabolism during exercise and recovery in patients with respiratory failure. *Thorax* **48**:486–90.

Toshima M.T., Kaplan, R.M., and Ries, A.L. (1990) Experimental evaluation of rehabilitation in chronic obstructive pulmonary disease: short term effects on exercise endurance and health status. *Health Psychol.* **9**:237–52.

Whipp, B.J., and Casaburi, R. (1994) Physical activity, fitness and chronic lung disease. In *Exercise, Fitness and Health* (eds C. Bouchard, R.J. Shephard, T. Stephens, J.R. Sutton and B.D. McPherson). Champaign, Illinois: Human Kinetics, pp. 749–61.

4b. Aerobic exercise training in patients with COPD

S.J. Singh

Department of
Respiratory Medicine
and Thoracic Surgery,
Glenfield Hospital,
Leicester

Practical Pulmonary Rehabilitation.
Edited by Mike Morgan and Sally Singh.
Published in 1997 by Chapman & Hall, London.
ISBN 0 412 61810 9.

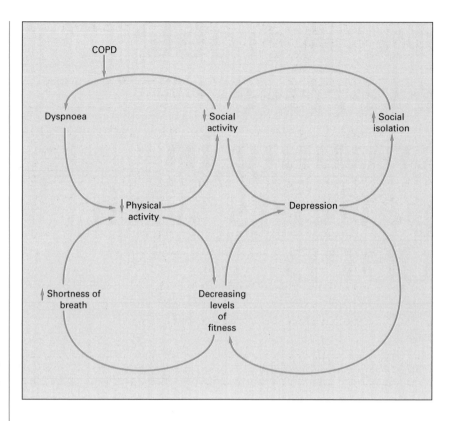

Fig. 4b.1 The vicious circle of chronic obstructive pulmonary disease (COPD).

The patient with chronic obstructive pulmonary disease (COPD) commonly presents to either the general practitioner or physician with the symptoms of breathlessness and/or exercise intolerance. In an attempt to offset these symptoms and declining functional capacity, exercise training must be considered. At present the exact mechanism by which patients improve their exercise tolerance is not fully understood. However, profound improvements in patients' performance are widely documented. Consequently, pulmonary rehabilitation has become a popular treatment option for those individuals who recognize the loss of function resulting from deconditioning. This disability is frequently accompanied by depression and social isolation (Fig. 4b.1). An element of exercise training is the foundation of most rehabilitation programmes.

There are numerous approaches to training; arguably the most important are discussed within this section of the book. The aim of this chapter is to identify possible aerobic training regimes. Aerobic (i.e. oxidative) training seeks to alter physiological mechanisms that allow the individual to sustain the particular activity for a longer period of time. Briefly, this method of training increases the capacity of the oxygen delivery systems allowing the individual an increased endurance time. The term fitness is often used alongside training but means something quite different: fitness refers to the persistent ability to perform moderate to vigorous exercise without undue fatigue.

Ventilatory response to exercise

If a patient with COPD is required to perform an incremental exercise test a point is rapidly reached when the ventilatory system is compromised. The elevated functional residual capacity (FRC) observed at rest is accentuated during exercise (increased expiratory time, increased frequency and activity of inspiratory muscles). This allows higher expiratory flow rates to be reached for the same driving pressure (due to the shift of the exercising flow/volume curve). Unfortunately, this increase in FRC becomes self-limiting as the load on the inspiratory muscles increases. In addition the pressures required to generate flow compromise the patency of the alveoli and airways. This increased load on the respiratory muscles predisposes to fatigue and, combined with muscle dysfunction, leads to limitation of exercise performance.

Limitations to exercise in patients with COPD

Exercise tolerance in patients with COPD is reduced. A number of reasons why patients experience this reduction have been reported, ranging from compromised gas exchange to cardiac limitation. However, the consensus of opinion suggests that the major limitation is related to abnormal mechanical characteristics of the respiratory system, i.e. an inability to increase ventilation to meet the demands of exercise. Evidence of a ventilatory limit to exercise is revealed when comparisons are made with normal individuals and patients with COPD. A sedentary male may reach a maximum ventilation (V_E) of 140 l, in sharp contrast to a patient's values. Values for patients' maximum V_E have been recorded as low as 26.9 l/min (Swinburn *et al.*, 1985). An alternative comparison with the norm can be made with regard to the maximum voluntary ventilation (MVV); in normal subjects the maximal exercise ventilation is around 70% of the MVV (Whipp and Pardy, 1986), whilst in COPD this value is commonly 100% (Jones *et al.*, 1971).

Cardiovascular factors appear to be relatively insignificant in limiting performance, and low maximal heart rates are consistently documented (Nery *et al.*, 1983). Patients do, however, present with an upwards shift of the oxygen consumption (V_{O_2})/heart rate slope – at a comparable V_{O_2} a patient with COPD will have a higher heart rate.

Recently attention has been directed towards studying latent cardiac abnormalities affecting exercise performance. Factors identified as limiting cardiac output were coexisting ischaemic heart disease (most patients with COPD are old and have smoked) and pulmonary hypertension (associated with structural abnormalities of the lung, compounded by hypoxic vasoconstriction; Wagner, 1992). It has also been documented that right ventricular function is decreased in this group of patients (Matthay *et al.*, 1992), but its contribution to exercise cessation is unclear.

The work of breathing has two main components: first, the work against the lung elasticity and second, the work performed in generating airflow, both of which are disturbed in patients with COPD (Beck *et al.*, 1991). This leads to an increase in the work of breathing. The significance of respiratory muscle fatigue in causing exercise intolerance is unclear, and discussed in Chapter 4c.

Until recently, peripheral muscle fatigue was overlooked as a limitation to exercise in patients with COPD. Killian *et al.* (1992) demonstrated that a substantial number of patients stopped exercising on a cycle ergometer because of leg pain. It remains to be confirmed whether this pattern would be repeated with treadmill walking, an activity which is more familiar to patients with COPD.

The perception of breathlessness is unique to each patient. The sensation is strongly influenced by the individual's psychological state at the time of assessment. Awareness of dyspnoea may itself limit exercise independently of any mechanical/physiological mechanisms. Altose (1985) proposes a variety of signals that may be responsible for mediating the sensation of breathlessness, including chemoreceptors in the blood and brain, mechanoreceptors in the thorax and outgoing central nervous system respiratory motor commands.

While the mechanism limiting exercise performance in patients with COPD is not fully understood, factors may include ventilation, circulation, ventilation/perfusion inequality, muscular and psychological reasons (Table 4b.1). A consensus of opinion exists that most patients have a ventilatory limit.

Response to aerobic training in patients with COPD

In normal individuals the response of aerobic training is thought to centre around the changes in the trained muscle (increases in the capillary network, mitochondrial density and concentration of the oxidative enzymes) and the cardiovascular system (increased stroke volume). The response observed in the patient is more controversial. A long-running hypothesis suggests that patients with COPD are unable to train sufficiently to induce a metabolic change in the exercising muscle, thus

Table 4b.1 What limits exercise in chronic lung disease?	
Maximal	*Endurance*
Lung mechanics	Lung mechanics
Lactic acidosis	Substrate availability
Arterial hypoxaemia	Motivation
Motivation	Poor coordination
Peripheral fatigue	
Poor coordination	

making it a more efficient user of the oxygen delivered. This is based on the observation that the majority of patients with COPD terminate an exercise test because of breathlessness and not local muscle fatigue. The direct muscle work by Belman and Kendregan (1981) is supportive of this theory. It should be noted, however, that the individuals trained initially at 33% of their maximal capacity and this of itself may have been an inadequate stimulus to provoke change.

Other workers dispute this lack of change (Casaburi *et al.*, 1991) and suggest that alternative physiological mechanisms can account for changes in exercise tolerance measured pre- and post-rehabilitation. It is proposed that patients with COPD require a low stimulus to provoke a conditioning response (Casaburi *et al.*, 1991) and second, patients can gain a beneficial effect due to the reduced ventilatory drive associated with a decrease in blood lactate concentrations. This is based on the assumption that patients with COPD performing an exercise test are likely to reach an anaerobic threshold (AT). This AT represents the threshold at which the oxidative metabolism is supplemented by anaerobic pathways; at the same time the production of lactate exceeds its breakdown and is a measurable metabolite of anaerobic metabolism. As a consequence of this increased lactic acid production, ventilation increases because of the need to clear the excess carbon dioxide (a byproduct of lactic acid breakdown). This has been well demonstrated by the work of Casaburi *et al.* (1989). The group demonstrated that patients with COPD able to exercise and achieve an AT were amenable to training. The patients responded to high-intensity aerobic training, measurable as a significant decrease in lactate production, V_E, etc. This study provides some support for a physiological response to training. Patessio *et al.* (1993a) speculate that only those patients able to produce a substantial lactate response post-exercise are likely to have reduced ventilatory requirements post-exercise training.

Physiology aside, alternative mechanisms commonly documented for this increase in exercise tolerance are desensitization to breathlessness, increased confidence and motivation and improved neuromuscular coordination.

Training regimens

Review of the recent literature reveals that there is no consensus of opinion about the length of the rehabilitation programme, the intensity or duration of the exercise component, or indeed, the type of exercise training. The variety of rehabilitation regimens is bewildering. However, there are certain core elements that should be common to all programmes that prescribe exercise. Most importantly, the exercise prescription should be individualized to suit each person's functional capacity. After this the prescription should define the duration, frequency, intensity and finally the progression (all of which will be discussed below).

What mode of exercise can be employed?

Walking and cycling are the activities most commonly prescribed for endurance (aerobic) training. In addition to these, swimming, running and some upper-limb exercises (e.g. upper-limb cycle ergometry) fall under the umbrella term aerobic exercise, although they are less frequently employed. It is well documented that the response to training is training specific. Therefore the mode of training should reflect the activities that the patient would perform regularly. There is some transference of effect when large muscle masses are exercised.

If the patient is to continue with exercise upon discharge from the programme, the exercise needs to be comfortable and accessible to the patient. This problem can be addressed in one of three ways. First, the patient could continue to attend the hospital to use the facilities in the gym to train; this would, however, have profound financial implications for the unit. Alternatively the individual could buy equipment for their home or, finally, be prescribed a mode of training that can be continued at home with no financial consequences for the patient. In the UK, it is therefore more practical to prescribe walking or stair-climbing as the aerobic activity. Cycling, although acceptable to the patient whilst in the gym, is likely to be extremely difficult to replicate at home.

Exercise prescription

Exercise prescription can either be based on the results of a laboratory-based exercise test or a field exercise test where some estimation of maximal capacity is secured. From either exercise test there are a combination of parameters that can be used to prescribe exercise (Fig. 4b.2).

Direct measures of peak oxygen consumption

A laboratory-based exercise test allows a precise prescription of exercise, commonly expressed as a percentage of the peak oxygen consumption (VO_{2peak}).

Few studies use the measurement of VO_{2peak} to prescribe exercise protocols (Casaburi *et al.*, 1991; Punzal *et al.*, 1993). Several studies incorporated the measurement of VO_{2peak} into their battery of pre- and post-rehabilitation studies. VO_{2peak} is considered to be the 'gold standard' measure of functional capacity. The paucity of data relating to this method of prescription possibly indicates the confusion as to the best way forward and second, the supervision required for this type of programme is potentially intense.

Lactate concentration measurements

An additional measure taken during a laboratory- or field-based exercise test is blood lactate concentrations. This method, available in some hospitals, allows the prescription of exercise to manipulate the lactate build-up and hence modify the increased demand on the ventilatory system. This method obviously relies on patients performing an exercise test to develop a significant increase in blood lactate concentrations. The data to support this are not conclusive.

Indirect measures of VO_2

It may be possible to use field exercise tests to estimate an individual's VO_{2peak} and from this point define an exercise intensity responding to the required level. The shuttle walking test exhibits a strong relationship with an individual's VO_{2peak} (Singh *et al.*, 1994). This may allow a reasonably accurate intensity of exercise, i.e. speed of walking, to be prescribed from the results of a field walking test. This could be further secured by calibrating it against either heart rate or perceived breathlessness (see below).

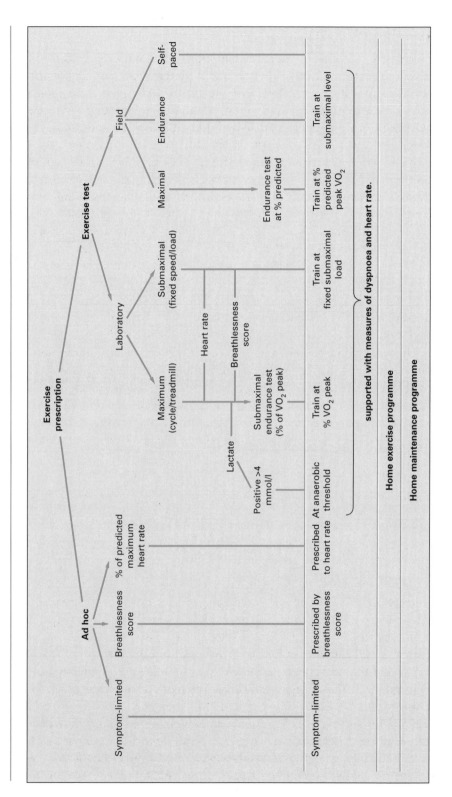

Fig. 4b.2 A potential mechanism to prescribe exercise for patients with chronic obstructive pulmonary disease.

Symptom-limited exercise training

A common approach to exercise training patients with COPD is to rely on the patient terminating the training regimen when suitably breathless (Sinclair and Ingram, 1980; Tydeman *et al.*, 1984). The perception of breathlessness differs from person to person and needs to be prescribed specifically to each patient. Scales used could be either the Borg score (Borg, 1982) or a visual analogue scale. The Borg breathlessness or perceived exertion score can be used simultaneously. The former is a 10-point categorical scale to describe symptoms, ranging from nothing at all to maximal. The exertion scale ranges from 6 to 20 with description provided at every odd number. The Borg responses to incremental exercise correspond closely with cardiorespiratory and metabolic indices. Therefore a Borg score can be used to establish an exercise intensity for aerobic training. In normal individuals it has been demonstrated that to exercise to an exertion rating of 12–13 (of the perceived exertion scale) a training load of approximately 60% of maximal heart rate is achieved. To exercise to 85% of maximum a rating of 16, 'hard to very hard', is suggested. Without access to sophisticated exercise-testing equipment it may be appropriate to train a patient with COPD between 3 and 5 (moderate to severe) on the Borg breathlessness score. The perception of breathlessness depends on the person and a patient may select an inappropriate response to train effectively. For these individuals prescription of exercise using these scales may be inappropriate or need modification.

Heart rate

In normal healthy individuals there is a linear relationship between heart rate and work load, thus making the prescription of exercise relatively straightforward. From a submaximal exercise test it is possible to extrapolate the work rate/heart rate relationship of that individual and thus estimate the maximal work intensity that coincides with the predicted maximal heart rate. From this point it is possible to calculate a training intensity that would equal, for example, 50–60% of the maximum (calculated as $210 - (0.65 \times age)$). This relationship is disturbed in patients with COPD. Although the relationship between work rate and heart rate is linear it is shifted upwards and to the left in patients with COPD. The maximal heart rate is likely to fall well below the predicted maximum. It is therefore invalid to assume that a true maximum can be predicted.

A maximal incremental exercise test allows the definition of the true symptom-limited maximal heart rate to be identified and exercise can be prescribed and monitored from this point. Monitoring can either be with a piece of simple equipment (sports tester PE3000) or taken by the patient. The monitoring of heart rate allows a discrete progression of exercise as the cardiovascular system responds to the exercise and the individual is able to exercise to a greater intensity for an equivalent heart rate. A summary of the options for exercise training and mechanisms to standardize these interventions is displayed in Figure 4b.2.

What makes an effective exercise regimen?

This question has puzzled those involved with rehabilitation for some time. Perhaps one of the most obvious reasons for this is the lack of convincing evidence documenting significant physiological changes in patients with COPD in response to endurance training. If, as has been suggested, the response is mediated primarily through psychosocial parameters resulting in a desensitization to breathlessness, then perhaps it doesn't really matter how the individuals are trained. The evidence suggests that it is important particularly to increase the capacity for the activities performed regularly.

There are certain components that need to be defined for an effective exercise programme including duration, frequency and intensity. The relative importance of each has not been convincingly identified; it would seem a reasonable assumption that there is considerable overlap in these components. Cardiovascular improvements can be defined as a product of the intensity and the duration of the exercise. Perhaps equally important but less often quoted are the severity of disability in the group and the enthusiasm of the patients and team of medical personnel monitoring the training component of the programme.

Intensity

Endurance training should be prescribed individually and according to the patient's functional capacity and limitations. Sadly, there is little unanimity over the optimum intensity of training for patients with COPD. The most frequently quoted threshold for training is in relation to the maximum oxygen consumption ($V_{O_{2max}}$), i.e. 50% of this maximal value. It has been demonstrated in healthy individuals that training at a walking speed equivalent to 50% of the $V_{O_{2max}}$ provokes a significant improvement in performance (Stensel *et al.*, 1992). It is suggested that a similar intensity may be appropriate for a population with COPD. In normal subjects it is well documented that the anaerobic threshold coincides with approximately 50% of the individual's $V_{O_{2max}}$. This threshold may well coincide with the training threshold in patients with COPD; more studies are required to examine this threshold for training and to reveal the relative importance of timing and intensity of training.

Recently it was demonstrated that individuals with COPD may be able to train at a higher percentage of their $V_{O_{2max}}$ (Punzal *et al.*, 1993). While such regimes appear to be successful, the results have to be balanced against a greater risk of injury and the implications of the increased supervision required. There is little agreement about the total amount of work done per session and the importance of intensity versus duration. If an individual works for a short time at a high intensity this would provoke a broadly similar physiological response to exercise maintained for longer but at a lower intensity. A substantial number of patients with COPD are unable to sustain activity even at a low intensity; for these individuals it is perhaps easier to increase the duration rather than the intensity. From our experience most individuals express a desire to improve their endurance capacity rather than complete a task quicker.

Should patients be categorized for training?

It has been proposed by Patessio *et al.* (1993b) that the prescription of exercise could be based upon the combined measures of resting lung function values, a significant blood lactate response and oxygen consumption. Yet it is agreed that measures of lung capacity do not relate well to an individual's ability to perform exercise. Individuals able to produce a lactate response during a maximal test are the one category of patients believed to accomplish a true physiological response and should be trained above this threshold level. Alternatively, those patients unable to mount a response and/or those with low forced expiratory volume in 1 s (FEV_1) values should train to a symptom-limited intensity, whilst the most disabled patient trains at a self-prescribed speed. The majority of programmes operating within the UK are unlikely to have the facility to measure blood lactate concentrations, therefore this type of discrimination is not possible. From our experience it is achievable and sensible to train a cross-section of patients together using a similar mode of training. Most importantly, all patients should be individually prescribed exercise. From this point, all patients can integrate successfully into a rehabilitation programme. There are very few individuals who cannot walk on a treadmill at an individually prescribed submaximal speed for even a short time; this could form the foundation of a training regimen.

Duration of the exercise session

Traditionally a pulmonary rehabilitation course allows an hour for exercise and a subsequent hour for education. The former contains a bout of endurance training, a warm-up (5–10 min) and a cool-down (5–10 min).

> ## Components of an effective training regimen
>
> Appropriate and individualized prescription of:
>   Duration
>   Frequency
>   Intensity
>   Progression
> Home exercise programme
> Maintenance programme

Alienation of the patient towards exercise has to be carefully circumnavigated. To this end, the initial training session should be within easy reach of the patient's capacity. Endurance training should aim to allow the patient to exercise for 20–30 min by the end of the course. Starting times for endurance walking/cycling may be as low as 1 min. Not all patients will be able to exercise for the allotted time. It is reasonable for the patient to complete two 10-min sessions or four 5-min sessions within the time. The importance of an individual prescription of exercise cannot be overemphasized.

A home exercise programme should be prescribed, identifying at least two additional sessions of endurance training at home. The duration of this exercise should mirror that achieved in the hospital.

Frequency

In the UK most rehabilitation programmes are outpatient based. This imposes obvious limitations on the frequency with which the group convene. Twice or three times a week is optimal, with the patient completing the same exercise at home on two occasions, if not more. The starting frequency is dictated in part by the individual's exercise tolerance. If this is severely diminished, it may be necessary to advise bouts of exercise on a daily basis. The completion of home exercise should be recorded on a diary card (Fig. 4b.3a). Most programmes run for between 6 and 8 weeks. The optimal response to an aerobic training programme usually occurs within 4–6 weeks in healthy individuals (American College of Sports Medicine, 1991). This is of course dependent upon the rate of progression of the individual. Someone with a low fitness level (typical of those recruited to a pulmonary rehabilitation programme) may take longer to realize the full benefit of an exercise programme.

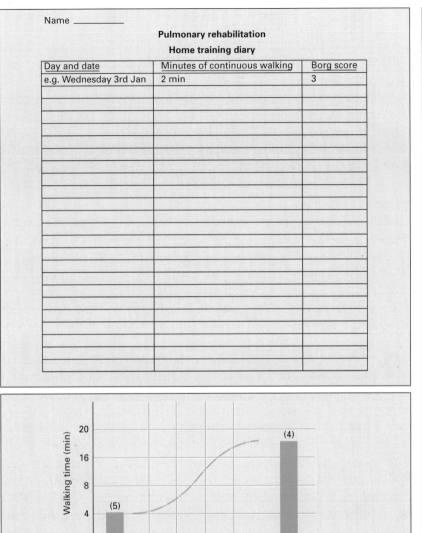

Name _____

Pulmonary rehabilitation

Home training diary

Day and date	Minutes of continuous walking	Borg score
e.g. Wednesday 3rd Jan	2 min	3

Fig. 4b.3(a) A diary card for the patient to record bouts of exercise performed away from the hospital.

Fig. 4b.3(b) Patient progression of home walking with treadmill measures of endurance capacity pre- and post-rehabilitation (Borg breathlessness scores in brackets).

Progression

The progression of the exercises should be carefully monitored and defined for the patient. The aim of the aerobic training is to allow the individual to increase the duration of exercise but maintain the intensity (resistance, walking, speed, stepping frequency). The rate of progression depends on the starting level of fitness, disease severity, age, motivation, compliance and goals. Initially the prescription should be modest to allow

93

adaptation to the rehabilitation programme and secure compliance. From here progression should be observed weekly, with target durations set for each patient. Often, after a couple of weeks in the programme, patients will take responsibility for their own progression. This is to be encouraged but the intensity of exercise needs to be carefully monitored. Often, once patients become accustomed to taking regular exercise the tendency is to increase the intensity (e.g. walking speed) as well as the duration. This often causes a plateau effect in the time achieved and simply requires a recalibration of walking speed (ideally on a treadmill).

Figure 4b.3b shows a typical response to a walking programme with pre- and post-treadmill endurance times documented on the chart as well as the home walking.

At the time of discharge it is important to identify a maintenance programme. This should be at the level attained at discharge, with advice to continue progressing if appropriate. Maintenance exercises should be performed at least three times a week.

Oxygen and exercise

The provision of oxygen may be necessary for those patients who demonstrate desaturation during exercise. Supplemental oxygen delivered during exercise reduces the respiratory rate, exercise ventilation and dyspnoea and increases the ability to perform exercise. Oxygen desaturation should be monitored during an exercise test, allowing an objective comparison to be made in the parameters defined above, when oxygen is administered. An oxygen saturation (SaO_2) of less than 88% is generally agreed to be the threshold measurement for the prescription of oxygen (these patients may or may not be prescribed long-term oxygen therapy at home). For patients between the values of 88 and 90% it may be necessary to consider supplemental oxygen if a decrease in breathlessness and an increase in work can be demonstrated.

At the time of writing the provision of ambulatory oxygen cylinders in the UK is confusing. Hospitals often have a supply of ambulatory oxygen cylinders (Fig. 4b.4) that allow the patient some degree of independence. At present it is difficult for patients to obtain these cylinders for home use. A further difficulty is that, because these cylinders contain compressed gas, they consequently have a short duration of oxygen. An alternative to compressed gas is liquid oxygen, commonly used in the rest of Europe and the USA. This system has advantages because it is lighter to carry and offers a longer period of oxygen to the patient. One disadvantage of ambulatory oxygen is, of course, the burden of the

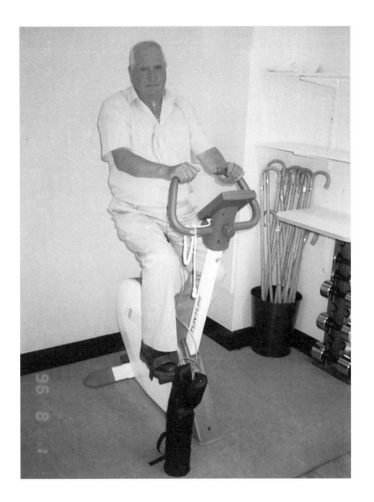

Fig. 4b.4 A portable oxygen cylinder can be supported by the patient or partner in an attempt to offset desaturation and improve exercise tolerance.

increased weight the patient is required to move with. Several studies suggest that this is a small price to pay for the increase in exercise tolerance.

Assessing the efficacy of the exercise programme

The most obvious demonstration of improved performance after rehabilitation is to perform an exercise test pre- and post-rehabilitation. Maximal oxygen uptake is quoted as an outcome measure for a rehabilitation programme. If a patient manifests a true ventilatory limit to maximal exercise performance it is well documented that maximal oxygen uptake rarely improves (Simpson *et al.*, 1992). On the other hand, if limitation to exercise is not ventilatory but is in fact peripheral, a

95

> ## Measuring the effectiveness of an exercise programme
>
> *Simple measures*
> Improved exercise tolerance
> (endurance > maximal)
> Decreased heart rate at equivalent work rate
> Decreased dyspnoea
> *Complex measures*
> Decreased ventilation at equivalent work rate
> Decreased blood lactate concentrations at equivalent work rate

Box 4b.2

heightened perception of breathlessness or psychological (motivation), then improvement in VO_{2peak} may well increase post-endurance training. A more sensitive method of assessing exercise tolerance is to perform a submaximal endurance test. This is designed to reflect the hypothesized physiological responses to endurance training and hence enhanced performance at submaximal loads.

Conclusion

Aerobic training can be a reasonably straightforward method of prescribing exercise for patients with COPD, requiring the minimum of equipment. Consequently it is a form of training accessible to all. In its most basic form it can be applied with just a measure of breathlessness (Borg, visual analogue score). Alternatively, if equipment is available, this method of training lends itself to a precise and scientific prescription of exercise.

References

Altose, D.M. (1985) Assessment and management of breathlessness. *Chest* **88**:77s–83s.

American College of Sports Medicine. (1991) *Guidelines for Exercise Testing and Prescription*, 4th edn. Philadelphia: Lea & Febiger.

Beck, C.K., Babb, T.G., Staats, B.A., and Hyatt, R.E. (1991) Dynamics of breathing during exercise. In: *Exercise, Pulmonary Physiology and Pathophysiology (Lung Biology in Health and Disease Series/52)* (eds B.J. Whipp and K. Wasserman). New York: Marcel Dekker, pp. 67–98.

Belman, M.J., and Kendregan, B.A. (1981) Exercise training fails to increase skeletal muscle enzymes in patients with chronic obstructive pulmonary disease. *Am. Rev. Respir. Dis.* **123**:256–61.

Borg, G.A.V. (1982) Psychophysical bases of perceived exertion. *Med. Sci. Sport Ex.* **14**:377–81.

Casaburi, R., Wasserman, K., Patessio, A. *et al.* (1989) A new perspective in pulmonary rehabilitation: anaerobic threshold as a discriminant in training. *Eur. Respir. J.* (suppl 7):618–23s.

Casaburi, R., Patessio, A., Ioli, F. *et al.* (1991) Reduction in exercise lactic acidosis and ventilation as a result of exercise training in patients with chronic lung disease. *Am. Rev. Respir. Dis.* **143**:9–18.

Jones, N.L., Jones, G., and Edwards, R.H.T. (1971) Exercise tolerance in chronic airways obstruction. *Am. Rev. Respir. Dis.* **103**:477–90.

Killian, K.J., Leblanc, P., Martin, D.H. *et al.* (1992) Exercise capacity and ventilatory, circulatory, and symptom limitation in patients with chronic airflow limitation. *Am. Rev. Respir. Dis.* **146**:935–40.

Matthay, R.A., Arroliga, A.C., Wiedermann, H.P. *et al.* (1992) Right ventricular function at rest and during exercise in chronic obstructive pulmonary disease. *Chest* **101**(suppl.):255s–62s.

Nery, L.E., Wasserman, K., French, W. *et al.* (1983) Contrasting cardiovascular and respiratory responses to exercise in mitral valve and chronic obstructive pulmonary diseases. *Chest* **83**:446–53.

Patessio, A., Casaburi, R., Carone, M. *et al.* (1993a) Comparison of gas exchange, lactate, and lactic acidosis thresholds in patients with chronic obstructive pulmonary disease. *Am. Rev. Respir. Dis.* **148**:622–26.

Patessio, A., Ioli, F., and Donner, C.F. (1993b) Exercise prescription. In: *Principles and Practice of Pulmonary Rehabilitation* (eds R. Casaburi and T. Petty). Philadelphia: WB Saunders.

Punzal, P.A., Reis, A.L., Kaplan, R.M., and Prewitt, L.M. (1993) Maximum intensity exercise training in patients with chronic obstructive pulmonary disease. *Chest* **100**:618–23.

Simpson, K., Killian, K., McCartney, N. *et al.* (1992) Randomised controlled trial of weight lifting in patients with chronic airflow limitation. *Thorax* **47**:70–5.

Sinclair, D.J.M., and Ingram, C.G. (1980) Controlled trial of supervised exercise training in chronic bronchitis. *Br. Med. J.* **i**:519–21.

Singh, S.J., Morgan, M.D.L., Hardman, A.E. *et al.* (1994) Comparison of oxygen uptake during a conventional treadmill test and the shuttle walking test in chronic airflow limitation. *Eur. Respir. J.* **7**:2016–20.

Stensel, D.J., Hardman, A.E., Brooke-Wavell, K. *et al.* (1992) The influence of brisk walking on endurance fitness in previously sedentary, middle aged men. *J. Physiol.* **446**:123p.

Swinburn, C.R., Wakefield, J.M., and Jones, P.W. (1985) Performance, ventilation and oxygen consumption in three different types of exercise tests in patients with chronic obstructive lung disease. *Thorax* **40**:581–6.

Tydeman, D.E., Chandeler, A.R., Graveling, B.M. *et al.* (1984) An investigation into the effects of exercise training on patients with chronic airways obstruction. *Physiotherapy* **70**:261–4.

Wagner, P.D. (1992) Ventilation–perfusion matching during exercise. *Chest* **101**:192s–8s.

Whipp, B.J., and Pardy, R.L. (1986) Breathing during exercise. In: *Handbook of Physiology Section 3. The Respiratory System*, vol. 3 (ed A.P. Fishman). Baltimore: Williams & Wilkins, pp. 605–29.

4c. Inspiratory muscle training

R.S. Goldstein

Department of
Respiratory Medicine,
University of Toronto,
Ontario, Canada

Practical Pulmonary Rehabilitation.
Edited by Mike Morgan and Sally Singh.
Published in 1997 by Chapman & Hall, London.
ISBN 0 412 61810 9.

Introduction

The role of ventilatory muscle training within the context of the clinical management of patients with altered ventilatory function remains unclear. One can predict that the ventilatory muscles will be unable to maintain their required or expected force (Edwards, 1978) if their rate of energy consumption exceeds that of their energy supply. Their energy consumption will be influenced by the work of breathing and the integrity of the contractile apparatus (Rochester and Arora, 1983) whereas their energy supply will be determined by the force and timing of muscle contraction and by the tissue oxygen delivery (Bellemare and Grassino, 1983). Training of the ventilatory muscles should follow the basic principles of training for any striated muscle with regard to the intensity and duration of the stimulus, the specificity of training and the reversibility of training. It is equally important to evaluate the outcome of training using appropriate clinical endpoints. This section will discuss the standard methods used for testing and training of the ventilatory muscles, the rationale for such training and the results of training programmes. It will end with conclusions for the clinician as to whether it is appropriate to include ventilatory muscle training as part of the clinical management of patients in whom the ventilatory system is involved.

Muscle strength

As in any striated muscle, the force of contraction is determined by:

1. The length of the muscle (length–tension relationship).
2. Whether or not the contraction is associated with shortening (force–velocity relationship).
3. The strength and frequency of stimulation (force–frequency relationship).
4. The integrity of the contractile apparatus (Rochester, 1988).

The length of the respiratory muscles varies with lung volume, with the inspiratory muscle contractile force being greatest between functional residual capacity (FRC) and residual volume (RV) and the expiratory muscle contractile force being greatest at total lung capacity (TLC). A bedside evaluation of a short sniff or a strong cough will reflect a subject's respiratory muscle strength and in many instances is all that is required for the health professional to evaluate respiratory muscle strength. The standardized laboratory method of evaluating strength is the one described by Black and Hyatt (1969) in which the subject is encouraged to make maximal efforts against a closed airway. More invasive measurements include ballooned catheter assessments of oesophageal (pleural) and gastric (abdominal) pressure and their difference, the transdiaphragmatic pressure (Pdi). The Pdi recorded during a sniff from FRC provides an accurate and reproducible measure of inspiratory strength (Miller *et al.*, 1985) and oesophageal pressure recorded during a cough reliably reflects expiratory muscle strength (Arora and Galt, 1981).

Recently, there has been considerable interest in bilateral simultaneous transcutaneous phrenic nerve stimulation in the assessment of diaphragmatic strength. The amplitude of the shock is monitored from the muscle mass action potential (M-wave) recorded with surface electrodes. A painless, accurate and non-invasive measure of diaphragmatic contractility can be achieved by measuring mouth pressure against an occluded airway during phrenic nerve twitch stimulation. With the glottis open and the airway closed at the mouth, mouth pressure is a good estimate of the overall pleural surface pressure change (Yan *et al.*, 1992).

Muscle endurance

Ventilatory muscle endurance will be determined by its fibre-type composition, the adequacy of its blood supply and the integrity of its contractile apparatus (Rochester, 1988). In addition, endurance will be influenced by the force and duration of contraction and the velocity of shortening during the contraction. Because the force of contraction is expressed in relationship to its maximal value, muscle strength will have an important influence on endurance.

Tests of endurance

Tests of endurance include hyperpnoea, resistive loading, threshold loading and maximal static contractions.

Hyperpnoea

The laboratory evaluation of endurance has included measurements of sustained ventilation and of sustained pressure. The simplest is the maximal voluntary ventilation (MVV), a brief (12- or 15-s, depending on the study) period during which the subject is encouraged to sustain maximum ventilation with no extrinsic ventilatory load. The test reflects voluntary neural drive, airway resistance and respiratory muscle strength (Aldrich *et al.*, 1982). In 1968, Tenney and Reese studied isocapnoeic hyperpnoea and reported that the logarithm of endurance time varied linearly (negative slope) with the percentage of maximal breathing capacity (MBC; 20-s MVV). They also reported that estimates of power of breathing against endurance time were consistent with a simple model in which energy is derived from a fixed finite store and from a steady supply. Subsequently, Leith and Bradley (1976) evaluated the influence of ventilatory muscle endurance using sustained isocapnoeic hyperpnoea and noted that the sustained ventilatory capacity when plotted against endurance time became asymptotic at approximately 80% of MVV. Studies among healthy volunteers, subjects with chronic obstructive pulmonary disease (COPD) and those with cystic fibrosis reported that their maximum sustained ventilatory capacity (MSVC) for 15 min was between 60 and 100% of their MVV (Keens *et al.*, 1978c).

Resistive loading

Measurements of endurance based on the time for which subjects could overcome alinear inspiratory resistive loads have become popular following a classic study by Roussos and Macklem (1977). In this study, healthy volunteers were invited to breathe to exhaustion against an alinear inspiratory resistance at a given predetermined transdiaphragmatic pressure which was measured with two balloons and displayed to the subject on an oscilloscope. At FRC the Pdi that could be generated indefinitely was approximately 40% of the Pdi_{max}, with contraction and relaxation times being relatively equal.

Given that the diaphragm contracts during inspiration, it should tire more rapidly if at any given tension the ratio of inspiratory time to the duration of the breathing cycle (Ti/Ttot) is increased. Bellemare and Grassino (1982) have pointed out that the duty cycle is an important component of inspiratory muscle endurance. They proposed a tension–time index for the diaphragm (TTdi) which incorporated both the pressure (Pdi/Pdi_{max}) and the duty cycle (Ti/Ttot). The TTdi in healthy volunteers becomes critical at about 0.15. This critical index of work is similar to the tensions known to cause blood flow limitation in other skeletal muscles. The physiological implication of this finding is that if the diaphragm is obligated to exceed its critical tension, its ability to perform work will be limited by its oxygen consumption during relaxation when blood flow is restored and it may fail.

Threshold loading

In 1982, Nickerson and Keens devised a method for measuring ventilatory muscle endurance as the sustainable inspiratory pressure (SIP), which is the highest pressure a subject can generate in each breath for 10 min. A weighted plunger was used as an inspiratory valve. This

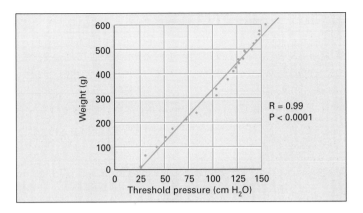

Fig. 4c.1 Relationship
between weight on plunger
and threshold mouth pressure.
The line of regression is
shown. From Nickerson and
Keens (1982), with
permission.

ensured that a minimum pressure was generated with each breath (Fig.
4c.1). In 15 healthy volunteers aged between 5 and 75 years, the SIP was
82 ± 6 (s.e.) cmH_2O or $68 \pm 3\%$ of their maximum inspiratory pressure.
Chen and Kuo (1989) tested 160 healthy volunteers using this technique
and reported that first, endurance was greater in men who were physically active than those who were sedentary; second, it was higher in men
than in women and third, that it decreased with age.

Maximal static contractions

A more recent approach to the measurement of respiratory muscle
endurance involves repeated maximal contractions against a closed
airway. This technique has the advantage of allowing respiratory muscles
to be compared with limb muscles under similar circumstances (Newell
et al., 1989) and has been reported in both healthy volunteers and in subjects with respiratory disease (Fig. 4c.2).

Histochemical composition

It has become clear that the performance of the respiratory muscles is
linked to their histochemical composition (Table 4c.1). This property of
all skeletal muscle is reflected in its fibre types. Generally, type I fibres
have a high oxidative capacity and a relatively low concentration of glycolytic enzymes. They are activated by smaller motor neurons recruited
early during the orderly recruitment of motor units and, although they
produce low levels of force relative to their cross-sectional area, they are
fatigue resistant. The time from the onset of contraction to peak tension
is slow and they are referred to as slow-twitch fibres. Type IIA muscle
fibres are intermediate in oxidative capacity, enzyme concentration and
fatigue resistance. Type IIB muscle fibres are low in oxidative capacity

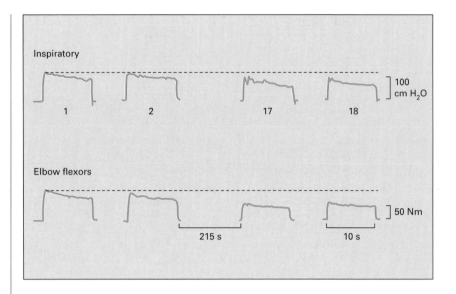

Fig. 4c.2 Records from a typical study in a control subject. Repeated maximal static contractions of the inspiratory muscles (upper panel) at functional residual capacity and of the elbow flexor (lower panel). The contractions lasted 10 s with rest intervals of 5 s (that is, a duty cycle of 67%). Note that the decline in peak and average sustained force was less for the inspiratory muscles than for the elbow flexors. From Newell *et al.* (1989), with permission.

Table 4c.1 Properties of muscle fibre types

| | Fibre type | | |
Characteristic	I	IIA	IIB
Twitch type	Slow	Fast	Fast
Colour	Intermediate	Red	White
Myosin ATPase activity	Low	High	High
Glycolytic capacity	Low	Intermediate	High
Oxidative capacity	High	High	Low
Mitochondrial density	High	High	Low
Endurance capacity	Excellent	Good	Poor

ATPase = Adenosine triphosphatase.
From Rochester (1988), with permission.

and have a high concentration of glycolytic enzymes. They are activated by larger motor neurons recruited later during the orderly recruitment of motor units and they fatigue rapidly. The time from the onset of contraction to peak tension is fast and they are referred to as fast-twitch fibres. In the diaphragm of normal adults, there are approximately 55%

type I fibres whereas premature infants who may be prone to muscle dysfunction have less than 10% (Keens *et al.*, 1978).

Rationale for training

The early studies of ventilatory muscle training were among healthy volunteers who, when encouraged to breathe to exhaustion (Bai *et al.*, 1984) at levels of ventilation close to their maximum, had measurable changes in the pressure–frequency relationship of their diaphragm, their maximum diaphragmatic pressure and their diaphragmatic electromyogram. However, such levels of ventilation are rarely encountered during day-to-day activities. When ventilatory muscle training has been applied among healthy volunteers in peak athletic condition (maximum oxygen consumption or $V_{O_{2max}} > 60\,\text{ml/kg}$) it did not influence $V_{O_{2max}}$ or endurance cycling at 90% of maximal power output (Fairbarn *et al.*, 1991).

In contrast, there are a variety of diseases in which the ventilatory muscles may influence gas exchange, the level of physical activity or the sensation of dyspnoea (Table 4c.2). Such limitations unquestionably

Table 4c.2 Diseases sometimes associated with respiratory muscle weakness	
Neurological diseases	Quadriplegia
	Myasthenia gravis
	Botulism
	Poliomyelitis
	Guillain–Barré syndrome
Muscle diseases	Myopathy (for example, steroids)
	Specific muscle enzyme deficiencies
Connective tissue diseases	Polymyositis
	Dermatomyositis
	Systemic lupus erythematosus
Endocrine disorders	Thyrotoxicosis
	Cushing's disease
Metabolic disorders	Hypophosphataemia
	Hypocalcaemia, hypomagnesaemia
	Metabolic alkalosis

From Pardy *et al.* (1981), with permission.

Table 4c.3 Effect of hyperpnoeic training on ventilatory muscles

| Reference | No. of subjects | Endurance | | | | Better than control subjects? |
		Duration	Frequency	Course	Response*	
Leith and Bradley (1976)	4 normal	20–30 min	5 weeks	5 weeks	19%	Yes
Keens *et al.* (1978c)	4 normal	25 min	5 weeks	4 weeks	22%	
	4 with cystic fibrosis	25 min	5 weeks	4 weeks	55%	Yes
Belman and Mittman (1980)	10 with COPD	30 min	5 weeks	6 weeks	33%	
Levine *et al.* (1986)	15 with COPD	15 min	5 weeks	6 weeks	41%	Yes
Ries and Moser (1986)	5 with COPD	30 min	5 weeks	6 weeks	16%	No

* Increase in maximum sustained ventilatory capacity.
COPD = Chronic obstructive pulmonary disease.
From Belman (1993), with permission.

influence quality of life and if muscle training were to result in a useful functional improvement it would be indicated as part of the management of these conditions.

Methods of ventilatory muscle training

As in the modalities of testing, training regimens have focused on repeated maximal inspiratory and expiratory efforts against a closed airway for strength training and isocapnoeic hyperpnoea, resistive and pressure threshold loads for endurance training. Isocapnoeic hyperpnoea has been shown to improve test function among healthy volunteers and subjects with cystic fibrosis and COPD (Table 4c.3). Leith and Bradley (1976) have shown that after 5 weeks of ventilatory muscle training subjects trained for strength increased their strength by 55% whereas those who trained for endurance increased their MSVC from 81% to 96% of their MVV (Table 4c.4). This very well-designed study emphasized the importance of the specificity of training and the importance of the stimulus being sufficiently high enough to effect training. The programme was one of training for 5 days a week for 5 weeks. Strength trainers performed repeated maximal static inspiratory and expiratory manoeuvres

Table 4c.4 Ventilatory muscle response to training

	Control group	Strength trainers	Endurance trainers
Strength at FRC			
PE_{max}	4 ± 6	57 ± 9	10 ± 9
PI_{max}	-2 ± 6	54 ± 16	9 ± 13
Lung volumes			
TLC	0.7 ± 1.3	4.6 ± 1.4	1.9 ± 0.8
VC	-0.3 ± 2.2	3.6 ± 0.8	3.1 ± 1.2
Sustained ventilatory capacity (% MVV)	4.5 ± 1.5	3.8 ± 1.5	15.5 ± 5.0
MVV 15 s	0.8 ± 4.0	2.0 ± 0.7	14 ± 4.7

FRC = Functional residual capacity; PE_{max} = maximal expiratory pressure; PI_{max} = maximal inspiratory pressure; TLC = total lung capacity; VC = vital capacity; MVV = maximum voluntary ventilation.
From Leith and Bradley (1976), with permission.

against obstructed airways and endurance trainers performed isocapnoeic hyperpnoea to exhaustion at levels of ventilation equivalent to 50% of MVV.

Alinear resistances have also been applied to the inspiratory muscles for training. Pardy *et al.* (1981) used a simple home programme in which subjects inspired for 30 min per day (in two 15-min sessions) against their critical inspiratory resistance while watching television or reading a book. At the end of 2 months of training, the critical resistance that could be tolerated by the subject had increased. Unfortunately, subjects often change their breathing strategy to one of slow, deep inspirations in order to tolerate more easily the inspiratory resistance. It is therefore essential that the breathing pattern be controlled during training.

Clanton *et al.* (1985) used the threshold load to train healthy volunteers and Goldstein *et al.* (1989) trained patients for 30 min twice each day for 4 weeks. Endurance time for a load set at 43% maximal inspiratory pressure increased by 7 min.

Response to training

Normal skeletal muscles will adapt to training provided that the appropriate stimulus is applied (Keens *et al.*, 1978; Faulkner, 1985). The basic principles of training are:

1. For muscle fibres to change structure and function, they must be stressed (overloaded) above a critical threshold.
2. Training is specific for the stimulus: strength training will increase fibre size (muscle hypertrophy) whereas endurance training will increase oxidative enzymes and mitochondrial density, myoglobin content and capillary density.
3. Training is reversible and the effects will be reduced (deconditioning) if the training ceases.

Ventilatory muscles will undergo extensive metabolic adaptation to chronically increased respiratory loads, presumably to optimize muscle performance (Keens *et al.*, 1978c; Farkas and Roussos, 1982). Training does not produce any major shifts in the proportion of slow-twitch and fast-twitch fibres in skeletal muscle. Muscle will also adapt to maximize its length–tension characteristics by altering the number of its sarcomeres (Farkas and Roussos, 1983). This process of adaptability of skeletal muscle may have an important bearing on the indications for training those patients with chronic respiratory disease. Keens *et al.* (1978c) noted that subjects with cystic fibrosis had a 36% higher ventilatory muscle endurance than did healthy volunteers and suggested that a process of adaptation to the chronic stress of breathing against high inspiratory loads had occurred. Similowski *et al.* (1991) evaluated the contractile properties of the human diaphragm during chronic hyperinflation and concluded that for the same lung volume the diaphragm function was as good as that measured in healthy volunteers.

Chronic obstructive pulmonary disease

There are good theoretical reasons to think that subjects with COPD may be expected to develop ventilatory muscle dysfunction. Their work and energy cost of breathing are substantially increased, whereas their capacity to endure such work may be diminished by mechanical and other influences. The main mechanical change is that of hyperinflation, which shortens the inspiratory muscles. This puts them at a disadvantageous position on their length–tension curve. Hyperinflation results in a marked decrease in the size of the zone of apposition between the costal fibres of the diaphragm and the ribcage (Tobin, 1988; Fig. 4c.3). The increased airway resistance results in an increased inspiratory load with each breath. COPD also influences the size and mass of the diaphragmatic muscle as part of the generalized weight loss that patients often experience. Another influence on ventilatory muscle function in COPD may be that of medications such as steroids which could further compromise muscle function. These influences on muscle func-

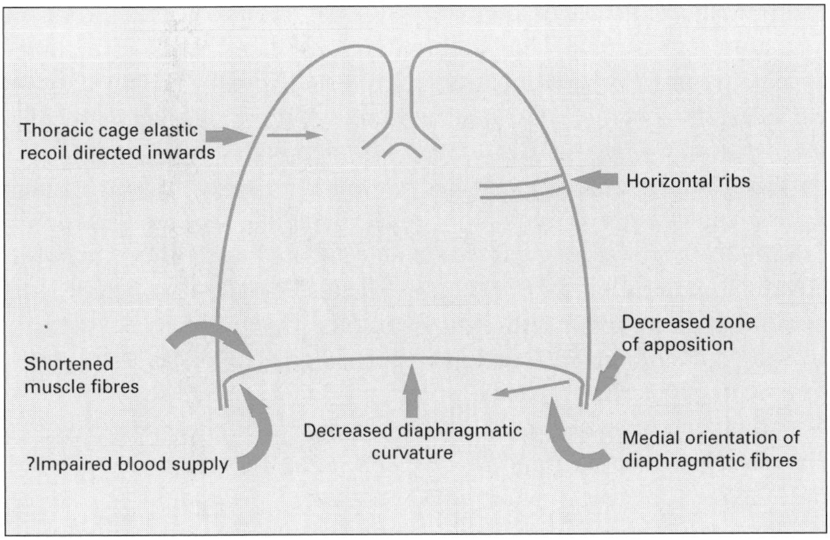

Labels in figure:
Thoracic cage elastic recoil directed inwards

Horizontal ribs

Decreased zone of apposition

Shortened muscle fibres

?Impaired blood supply

Decreased diaphragmatic curvature

Medial orientation of diaphragmatic fibres

Fig. 4c.3 The detrimental effects of hyperinflation on respiratory muscle function. From Tobin (1988), with permission.

tion may be closely linked to dyspnoea and to limitations in exercise performance.

Since the sensation of dyspnoea is related to the percentage of the maximum inspiratory pressure developed with each breath, it is possible that strengthening the inspiratory muscles may decrease dyspnoea. Strengthening of expiratory muscles may assist with secretion clearance. Endurance training might result in an increased capacity for higher levels of ventilation (such as in physical exercise) or for sudden increases in resistive loads (such as in infectious exacerbations). There is some preliminary evidence to suggest that inspiratory resistive training may assist those with chronic respiratory failure in being weaned from mechanical ventilation by providing brief periods of fatiguing exertion alternating with periods of complete rest (Aldrich, 1989). Thus subjects with COPD (bronchitis, emphysema, asthma, cystic fibrosis, bronchiectasis) could, at least in theory, benefit from training.

Results of training programmes

A very large number of studies have evaluated the influence of ventilatory muscle training. To summarize these studies, it appears as though subjects can be trained to improve their performance as measured by a particular test of endurance which is specific to the training modality. The evidence that such training results in functionally useful changes remains equivocal (Belman, 1993). Smith *et al.* (1992) reviewed 73 articles from a computerized bibliographic database and identified 17 rele-

vant randomized trials of ventilatory muscle training in chronic airflow
limitation. The authors combined effect sizes across studies (the difference between treatment and control groups divided by the pooled standard deviation of the outcome measure). A primary analysis of these
results showed that only MVV was associated with a significant *P* value
for the effect size. A secondary analysis was undertaken in which studies
were included only if ventilatory muscle training was associated with
control of the breathing pattern and compared with those in which
breathing pattern had not been controlled. The authors concluded that
respiratory muscle strength and endurance will improve but with no
associated alterations in functional exercise capacity or laboratory measurements of exercise capacity.

In their very thorough meta-analysis, Smith and colleagues (1992) did
not distinguish between trials comparing inspiratory muscle training
(IMT) alone and trials in which IMT was applied as an adjunct to exercise
training. Conceivably, the effects might be different depending on the
study design. Weiner *et al.* (1992a) added IMT to general exercise reconditioning (GER) in 12 patients (group A). In another 12 patients sham
training was added to exercise reconditioning (group B), while a further
12 patients acted as controls. Group A improved inspiratory muscle
strength and endurance. Both group A and group B improved walking
distance and submaximal exercise, although the improvements were
greater in group A than in group B. Wanke *et al.* (1994) randomized 21
patients to receive IMT in addition to cycle exercise training for 8 weeks.
Inspiratory muscle performance improved in those in whom the inspiratory muscles were trained but not in the control group. Both training
regimens increased maximal power output and VO_{2max} but the improvements were significantly greater in those with IMT. Both of the above
groups concluded that IMT intensified the beneficial effects of exercise
training.

In contrast, Berry *et al.* (1996) randomized 8 patients to GER plus IMT,
9 patients to GER alone and 8 patients to a control group. All patients
exercised three times per week for 12 weeks. The 12-min walk was
greater in the GER + IMT and GER groups than in the controls. Dyspnoea
during exercise did not differ from control. The authors concluded that
IMT conferred no additional benefit over GER on exercise performance
or on dyspnoea during exercise.

Although most of the above studies have involved subjects with
chronic bronchitis and emphysema, ventilatory muscle function has been
improved among subjects with cystic fibrosis (Keens *et al.*, 1978c; Asher
et al., 1982). Of interest, Keens *et al.* were able to induce changes in ventilatory muscle endurance of equivalent magnitude to that of endurance
training in 7 subjects who participated in a 4-week physical activity training programme consisting of 90 min/day swimming and canoeing.

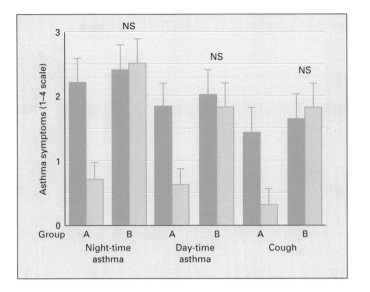

Fig. 4c.4 Diary-card data for asthma symptoms judged by the patients on a scale from 0, no symptoms to 4, very severe symptoms before and during the last 2 weeks of training. Open bars = before training; filled bars = after training. Values are mean ± s.e.m. From Weiner *et al.* (1992a), with permission.

Weiner *et al.* (1992b) described the results of IMT among 15 asthmatics compared with 15 control subjects. Subjects reported improvements in several indices of asthma in association with improvements in strength and endurance, including a reduction in the amount of inhaled β_2-agonists (Fig. 4c.4).

Non-obstructive ventilatory diseases

Although a variety of other conditions have been associated with ventilatory muscle weakness (Table 4c.2), there have been few studies evaluating the role of ventilatory muscle training for individuals with such conditions. An early study reported by Gross *et al.* (1980) concerned 6 chronic quadriplegics. Following IMT 30 min daily, 6 days a week, with loads sufficient to induce the electromyogram changes of fatigue, a significant increase in maximal inspiratory pressure and in critical inspiratory mouth pressure was noted. Whether such training protects against the clinical sequelae of an acute respiratory tract infection is unknown and has not been explored further. Ventilatory muscle training in tetraplegics has resulted in only small changes in their peak expiratory flow. In patients with neuromuscular disease, strength and endurance can be improved by training but the influence of such training on exercise tolerance, coughing and talking remains to be explored.

111

Outstanding issues

The above studies of ventilatory muscle training raise a number of interesting issues:

1. The evidence that physical exercise is associated with ventilatory muscle dysfunction rests on a few uncontrolled studies involving a small number of subjects.
2. Very few studies have measured dyspnoea or quality of life before and after ventilatory muscle training (Patessio *et al.*, 1989).
3. The role of expiratory muscle training has been relatively unexplored. Studies among healthy volunteers have confirmed that during exercise and during inspiratory resistive loading, the expiratory muscles are increasingly activated and there may be changes in the power spectrum of their electromyogram (Suzuki *et al.*, 1992).
4. Although harder to evaluate than strength or endurance training, improvements in the coordination of respiratory muscle function may be of benefit to some patients. Whole-body exercise may improve neuromuscular coordination and the efficiency of breathing. Pursed-lip breathing may minimize lung hyperinflation and diaphragmatic and abdominal breathing may reduce dyspnoea. The role of training coordination may be complementary to whole-body exercise and to specific training of the ventilatory muscles.

Conclusion

The subject of ventilatory muscle training is a fascinating study of the application of principles of training any striated muscle to the muscles of the ventilatory system. Training for strength and endurance has been achieved in healthy subjects and in those with chronic airflow limitation but only a few studies are available that describe the influence of training in other conditions. When training has occurred, the evidence that it results in changes that are functionally useful is at best equivocal. Training has generally focused on the muscles of inspiration and there is little information on the effect of expiratory muscle training. Natural adaptations of the muscles of respiration might militate against the need for training by maximizing their function against chronically increased loads. The design of training programmes must take into consideration an adequate training stimulus in terms of both intensity and duration and must control for the pattern of breathing. Although there is considerable potential for research that might identify the appropriate population for training, the best modality of training and the role of training within the context of other modalities of rehabilitation, there is insufficient evidence to justify the use of ventilatory muscle training in the clinical management of patients with chronic respiratory conditions.

References

Aldrich, T.K. (1989) The patient at risk of ventilator dependency. *Eur. Respir. J.* **2**:645s–51s.

Aldrich, T.K., Arora, N.S., and Rochester, D.F. (1982) The influence of airway obstruction and respiratory muscle strength on maximal voluntary ventilation in lung disease. *Am. Rev. Respir. Dis.* **126**:195–9.

Arora, N.S., and Galt, J. (1981) Cough dynamics during progressive expiratory muscle weakness in healthy curarized subjects. *J. Appl. Physiol.* **51**:494–8.

Asher, M.I., Pardy, P.L., Coates, A.L. *et al.* (1982) The effects of inspiratory muscle training in patients with cystic fibrosis. *Am. Rev. Respir. Dis.* **126**:855–9.

Bai, T.R., Rabinovitch, B.R., and Pardy, R.L. (1984) Near maximal voluntary hyperpnea and ventilatory muscle function. *J. Appl. Physiol.* **57**:1742–8.

Bellemare, F., and Grassino, A. (1982) Evaluation of human diaphragm fatigue. *J. Appl. Physiol.* **53**:1196–1206.

Bellemare, F., and Grassino, A. (1983) Force reserve of the diaphragm in patients with chronic obstructive pulmonary disease. *J. Appl. Physiol.* **55**:8–15.

Belman, M.J. (1993) Ventilatory muscle training and unloading. In: *Principles and Practice of Pulmonary Rehabilitation* (eds R. Casaburi and T.L. Petty). Philadelphia: WB Saunders.

Belman, M.J., and Mittman, C. (1980) Ventilatory muscle training improves exercise capacity in chronic obstructive pulmonary disease patients. *Am. Rev. Respir. Dis.* **121**:273–80.

Berry, M.J., Adair, N.E., Sevensky, K.S. *et al.* (1996) Inspiratory muscle training and whole body reconditioning in chronic obstructive pulmonary disease. *Am. J. Respir. Crit. Care Med.* **153**:1812–16.

Black, L.F., and Hyatt, R.E. (1969) Maximal respiratory pressures: normal values and relationship to age and sex. *Am. Rev. Respir. Dis.* **99**:696.

Chen, H.I., and Kuo, C.S. (1989) Relationship between respiratory muscle function and age, sex and other factors. *J. Appl. Physiol.* **66**:943–8.

Clanton, T.L., Dixon, G., Drake, J. *et al.* (1985) Inspiratory muscle conditioning using a threshold loading device. *Chest* **87**:62–6.

Edwards, R.H.T. (1978) Physiological analysis of skeletal muscle weakness and fatigue. *Clin. Sci. Mol. Med.* **54**:463–70.

Fairbarn, M.S., Coutts, K.C., Pardy, R.L., and McKenzie, D.C. (1991) Improved respiratory muscle endurance of highly trained cyclists and the effects on maximal exercise performance. *J. Sports Med.* **12**:66–70.

Farkas, G.A., and Roussos, C.D. (1982) Adaptability of the hamster diaphragm to exercise and/or emphysema. *J. Appl. Physiol.* **53**:1263–72.

Farkas, G.A., and Roussos, C.D. (1983) Diaphragm in emphysematous hamsters: sarcomere adaptability. *J. Appl. Physiol.* **54**:1635–40.

Faulkner, J.A. (1985) Structural and functional adaptations· of skeletal muscle. In: *Thorax* (eds C. Roussos and P.T. Macklem). New York: Marcel Dekker, pp. 1324–52.

Goldstein, R.S., De Rosie, J., Long, S. *et al.* (1989) Applicability of a threshold loading device for inspiratory muscle testing and training in patients with COPD. *Chest* **96**:564–71.

Gross, D., Ladd, H.W., Riley, E.J. *et al.* (1980) The effect of training on strength and the endurance of the diaphragm in quadriplegia. *Am. J. Med.* **68**:27–35.

Keens, T.G., Bryan, A.C., Levison, H., and Ianuzzo, C.D. (1978a) Developmental pattern of muscle fibre types in human ventilatory muscles. *J. Appl. Physiol.* **44**:909–13.

Keens, T.G., Chen, V., Patel, P. *et al.* (1978b) Cellular adaptations of the ventilatory muscles to a chronic increased respiratory load. *J. Appl. Physiol.* **44**:905–8.

Keens, T.G., Krastins, I.R.B., Wanamaker, E.M. *et al.* (1978c) Ventilatory muscle endurance training in normal subjects and patients with cystic fibrosis. *Am. Rev. Respir. Dis.* **116**:853–60.

Leith, D.E., and Bradley, M. (1976) Ventilatory muscle strength and endurance training. *J. Appl. Physiol.* **41**:508–16.

Levine, S., Weiser, P., and Gillen, J. (1986) Evaluation of ventilatory muscle endurance training program in the rehabilitation of patients with COPD. *Am. Rev. Respir. Dis.* **133**:400–6.

Miller, M.J., Moxham, J., and Green, M. (1985) The maximal sniff in the assessment of diaphragm function in man. *Clin. Sci.* **69**:91–7.

Newell, S.Z., McKenzie, D.K., and Gandevia, S.C. (1989) Inspiratory and skeletal muscle strength and endurance and diaphragmatic activation in patients with chronic airflow limitation. *Thorax* **44**:903–12.

Nickerson, B.G., and Keens, T.G. (1982) Measuring ventilatory muscle endurance in humans as sustainable inspiratory pressure. *J. Appl. Physiol.* **52**:768–72.

Pardy, R.L., Rivington, N., Despas, P.J., and Macklem, P.T. (1981) The effects of respiratory muscle training on exercise performance in chronic airflow limitation. *Am. Rev. Respir. Dis.* **123**:426–33.

Patessio, A., Rampulla, C., Fracchia, C. *et al.* (1989) Relationship between perception of breathlessness and inspiratory resistive loading: report on a clinical trial. *Eur. Respir. J.* **2**:587s–91s.

Ries, A.L., and Moser, K.M. (1986) Comparison of isocapnic ventilation and walking exercise training in pulmonary rehabilitation. *Chest* **90**:285–9.

Rochester, D.F. (1988) Tests of respiratory muscle function. *Clin. Chest Med.* **9**:249–61.

Rochester, D.F., and Arora, N.S. (1983) Respiratory muscle failure. *Med. Clin. North Am.* **67**:573–97.

Roussos, C.S., and Macklem, P.T. (1977) Diaphragmatic fatigue in man. *J. Appl. Physiol.* **43**:189–97.

Similowski, T., Sheng Yan, M.D., Gauthier, A.P. *et al.* (1991) Contractile properties of the human diaphragm during chronic hyperinflation. *N. Engl. J. Med.* **325**:917–23.

Smith, K., Cook, D., Guyatt, G.H. *et al.* (1992) Respiratory muscle training in chronic airflow limitation: a meta-analysis. *Am. Rev. Respir. Dis.* **145**:533–9.

Suzuki, S., Suzuki, J., Ishii, T. *et al.* (1992) Relationship of respiratory effort sensation to expiratory muscle fatigue during expiratory threshold loading. *Am. Rev. Respir. Dis.* **145**:461–6.

Tenney, S.M., and Reese, R.E. (1968) The ability to sustain great breathing efforts. *Respir. Physiol.* **5**:187–201.

Tobin, M.J. (1988) Respiratory muscles in disease. In: *Clinics in Chest Medicine* (ed M.J. Belman). pp. 263–86.

Wanke, T., Formanek, D., Lahrmann, H. *et al.* (1994) Effects of combined inspiratory muscle and cycle ergometer training on exercise performance in patients with COPD. *Eur. Respir. J.* **7**:2205–11.

Weiner, P., Azgad, Y., Ganam, R., and Weiner, M. (1992a) Inspiratory muscle training in patients with bronchial asthma. *Chest* **102**:1357–61.

Weiner, P., Azgad, Y., and Ganam R. (1992b) Inspiratory muscle training combined with general exercise reconditioning in patients with COPD. *Chest* **102**:1351–6.

Yan, S., Gauthier, A., Similowski, T. *et al.* (1992) Evaluation of human diaphragm contractility using mouth pressure twitches. *Am. Rev. Respir. Dis.* **145**:1064–9.

4d. Isolated muscle training in respiratory rehabilitation

D.G. Stubbing

Department of
Medicine, McMaster
University, Hamilton,
Ontario, Canada

Practical Pulmonary Rehabilitation.
Edited by Mike Morgan and Sally Singh.
Published in 1997 by Chapman & Hall, London.
ISBN 0 412 61810 9.

Introduction

Pulmonary impairment in the presence of chronic airflow limitation results in disability due to breathlessness. For individual patients this may be troublesome when trying to walk or undertake activity but it may also be problematic for tackling specific chores required for self-care or daily life. Studies have shown that peripheral muscle strength is also impaired in the presence of airflow limitation (Allard *et al.*, 1989) and that oxidative enzyme activity is reduced (Maltais *et al.*, 1996). These changes account for some of the disability that is present. Both of these abnormalities can be improved by a training programme with improvement in disability and quality of life.

Exercise training has become an integral part of the rehabilitation of the patient with chronic airflow limitation but general exercising training may not be applicable to the most severely disabled because the metabolic demand of a general exercise regimen may be too demanding for their ventilatory capabilities. General training may also not be applicable for aiding the performance of specific tasks, e.g. those requiring upper-extremity activity. In these situations isolated muscle training may be an appropriate method to achieve the goals of improving task performance and decreasing disability. This should reduce handicap and improve quality of life.

Isolated muscle training is taken to be not only the training of a specific muscle but also the training of a select group of muscles, which is usually aimed at aiding the performance of individual tasks. Simpson *et al.* (1992) trained several individual muscle groups for increasing strength and looked at both specific and general outcomes, whereas others have studied the effect of upper-extremity exercise training on specific outcomes related to arm activity. Although leg cycling exercise trains primarily the lower limbs for the tasks they perform, this section will not try to cover the effects as this is the mode usually adopted for general training. Similarly, inspiratory muscle training is discussed in a separate section (Chapter 4c), even though it is really isolated muscle group training.

Rationale for upper-extremity training

Once it was recognized that exercise training was the best way to decrease disability in patients with irreversible chronic airflow limitation, the thought of training upper extremities specifically for the tasks they perform was entertained. It was recognized that patients experienced what appeared to be an inordinate degree of breathlessness for the magnitude of the work when using arms compared to legs. The breathlessness is related to the metabolic demand of the task, plus the metabolic activity required to overcome gravity. This is aggravated by respiratory muscle dysfunction with upper-extremity activity as some of the chest wall muscles are involved in both respiration and arm activities.

Respiratory response to arm activity

The major reason for considering isolated muscle training for upper extremities is because of the frequent need to meet the ventilatory requirement of specific tasks using the arms. Martinez *et al.* (1991) studied the respiratory response to arm activity in 20 patients with severe airflow limitation (mean forced expiratory volume in 1 s or FEV_1 0.99 l) sitting either with the arms at the side or elevated to 90°. Arm elevation was accompanied by a 20% increase in oxygen consumption ($P < 0.01$) and a 23% increase in carbon dioxide production ($P < 0.01$) which resulted in an increase in minute ventilation of 18%. This was achieved through increases in both inspiratory and expiratory muscle activity. Dolmage *et al.* (1993) showed similar results with unsupported arm activity resulting in a 36% increase in oxygen consumption and a 35% increase in carbon dioxide production. However, when the elevated arms were supported in a sling (to counteract the effects of gravity) there was no significant change in any respiratory parameter. These studies indicate the magnitude of the respiratory response required as a result of the increased ventilatory demands of simple arm activity.

The symptoms which result from the respiratory response to upper-extremity exercise are aggravated or magnified by the effect of arm activity on respiratory muscle function. Celli *et al.* (1986) assessed respiratory muscle use with unsupported arm activity and showed that the ventilatory load was shifted more to the diaphragm and away from the accessory muscles and inspiratory ribcage muscles when the shoulder girdle was used for arm activity. In patients with chronic airflow limitation who rely on these accessory muscles even for resting ventilation, because of the effects of hyperinflation on the diaphragm, arm activity has a greater effect than in normal people.

Specificity of training

A second reason for using upper-extremity exercise training is because training is specific to the muscle groups involved. Although exercise training is not task specific (in other words, cycle training can improve walking), leg training is specific for leg muscle activity and arm training specific to upper-extremity activity.

Belman and Kendregan (1981) studied 15 individuals with airflow limitation. Seven underwent leg training and 8 arm training. A training period of 6 weeks included two 20-min sessions four times weekly with increasing workload and increasing duration of sessions up to 20 min. In those individuals who showed improvements, arm endurance increased only in the arm-trained group ($P < 0.01$) and leg endurance increased only in the leg-trained group ($P < 0.05$).

Specificity of muscle group training is also supported by Lake *et al.* (1990) who undertook a randomized controlled study in 28 patients with mean FEV_1 1.0 l and age 65.7 years. A control group was compared with three exercise groups, one of which undertook upper-limb training alone, one of which undertook lower-limb training alone and a third group which undertook combined upper- and lower-limb training. The study lasted 8 weeks, with three 1-h supervised sessions per week. Upper-limb training involved 20 min on a circuit with arm ergometry, throwing a ball, moving arms on a wire above the horizontal, transferring a bean bag over the head and a series of exercises with ropes and pulleys. Forty-second interventions were interspersed with 20-s rests. Lower-limb training was walking for 20 min and the combined group undertook both activities. The results showed an increase in 6-min walking distance only in the group that undertook leg training or combined training. An increase in maximum workload on the arm ergometer was only seen in those who undertook arm training or the combined training. In particular, there was no improvement in arm endurance with isolated leg training.

Upper-extremity training in rehabilitation

There have been several studies that assess the role of using upper-extremity training as part of a general rehabilitation programme. Ries *et al.* (1988) studied 45 subjects entering a 6-week rehabilitation programme. Only 28 subjects completed the study, 11 of whom were in a control group receiving the standard programme. Eight subjects were randomized to a programme of rehabilitation plus high-intensity upper-extremity exercise and 9 to the rehabilitation programme accompanied by low-intensity upper-extremity exercise. The specific arm training involved a series of exercises with weights added as tolerated and increasing repetitions over the course of the study. Although all three groups showed improvement, only those trained for upper extremities showed increases in upper-extremity performance. The most marked improvements in arm endurance and maximum workload occurred in the group that undertook high-intensity training.

Supported versus unsupported arm training

Couser *et al.* (1993) assessed the effect of upper-extremity training in 14 individuals in a rehabilitation programme who undertook a combination of leg cycling, supported arm exercise with arm ergometry and unsupported arm exercise with dowels and weights. They assessed the changes in oxygen consumption, carbon dioxide production and respiration during 2 min of unsupported arm elevation before and after the training periods. The training programme resulted in a 10% fall in minute ventilation ($P < 0.01$) at the end of 2 min of arm elevation, due to a 7% reduction in oxygen consumption ($P < 0.05$) and a 12% reduction in carbon dioxide production ($P = 0.01$). Symptoms related to task performance and quality of life were not reported.

Martinez *et al.* (1993) performed a similar study to assess the relative value of supported versus unsupported arm training. Forty patients in a rehabilitation programme involving general exercises plus respiratory muscle training were randomized to receive either supported or unsupported arm training in addition. Supported arm exercises were performed on an arm ergometer with the workload and duration of exercise increasing weekly to 15 min. Unsupported arm exercises involved holding a wooden dowel and performing shoulder flexion, shoulder circles, shoulder and elbow flexion and extension, elbow flexion and extension, and horizontal abduction and adduction. Endurance was increased in 30-s increments up to $3^{1}/_{2}$ min for each exercise, after which weights were added. Twelve-minute walking distance, cycle endurance and respiratory muscle strength improved in both groups ($P = $ not significant). Arm endurance on the ergometer increased in both groups but the measurement of endurance for unsupported arm activity increased more in those trained with unsupported arm exercises ($P < 0.002$). More importantly, the metabolic requirements of arm elevation only decreased in those who undertook unsupported arm exercise training ($P = 0.02$) and not in those who undertook the supported training programme ($P = 0.2$).

Strength training

Almost all of the studies of isolated muscle training have looked specifically at upper-extremity exercise. The exercises performed were a combination of weights, for strength training, and endurance training in addition to usual warm-ups and cool-downs. These studies assessed changes in task performance for the specific muscles trained. Simpson *et al.* (1992), however, studied weight training for both upper and lower limbs with outcome measures of change in muscle strength as well as change in disability, handicap and quality of life. Thirty-four patients,

121

44% of whom were female, with severe airflow limitation were stratified based on pulmonary impairment and oxygen status and then randomized to either a control group or a weight-training group. The control group attended at the beginning and end of the study for outcome measures. The intervention group participated in weight-training exercises using single-arm curl, single-knee extension and single-leg press on a Global Gym apparatus.

Initial assessment determined the maximum weight, for each of these exercises, which the subject could lift once. Training began using 50% of the maximum weight with 10 repetitions for each exercise, repeated three times, so that 30 repetitions of each were performed. The study lasted 8 weeks with three training sessions per week. As strength improved, maximum weight lifted was reassessed and training weight appropriately increased.

The training group showed a significant improvement in strength in all three muscle groups trained ($P < 0.01$) which was not seen in the control group. The maximum weight lifted for single-arm curl increased 33%, for single-knee extension increased 44% and for single-leg press increased 16%. Disability was assessed by exercise performance and improved only in the treatment group. Leg endurance, assessed by cycle endurance time at 80% of the initial maximum power output, increased in the treatment group but not in the control group. Cycle endurance was 518 s at the start of the study and increased to 898 s after weight training ($P < 0.01$). Similar values for the control group were 506 and 479 s respectively. In the intervention group 6-min walking distance showed a positive trend towards improvement but the change was not statistically significant. Walking distance increased from 391 ± 22.5 m to 427 ± 27 m. The control group did not change their walking distance: 369 ± 32 m at the initial assessment and 376 ± 32 m at the end of the study. As the sample size is small the lack of a significant change may represent a type II error. Unfortunately, measurements of task performance for the upper extremities were not made.

This study also assessed quality of life using the Chronic Respiratory Disease Questionnaire (Guyatt *et al.*, 1987). No changes were found in the control group but in the treatment group there were significant improvements in quality of life scores in the domains of dyspnoea ($P < 0.01$), fatigue ($P < 0.05$) and mastery ($P < 0.01$).

Weight-lifting training is of interest in chronic airflow limitation not only because it has been shown to be effective but because authors have shown excellent compliance. Ries *et al.* (1988) in their study reported compliance greater than 90% with the resistance training used for upper-extremity exercise. Their patients tended to prefer to increase resistance rather than the number of repetitions which were being performed. Simpson *et al.* (1992) also found excellent compliance, with more than

90% of scheduled sessions being attended by the individuals. This might be explained by the relative ease of the training sessions in the patients who found that the weight-training sessions did not cause undue breathlessness. Many patients with severe airflow limitation, however, have difficulty achieving a level of exercise on a cycle ergometer or treadmill which results in a true training effect because symptoms become limiting.

Practical application of isolated muscle training

Upper-extremity exercise

Upper-extremity exercise should become an integral part of the exercise component for all patients entering a respiratory rehabilitation programme. Allard *et al.* (1989) showed that in the presence of chronic airflow limitation peripheral muscle strength is reduced in both upper- and lower-extremity muscle groups. This, combined with the need to overcome gravity and the impairment of respiratory muscles which also occurs, probably accounts for the severity of the symptoms which patients recognize when they perform tasks using the arms. Arm exercise has been shown to improve arm performance, with unsupported exercises or high-intensity exercise having the greatest effect.

Training sessions should be similar to those used for leg muscles. Optimal frequency and duration are not perfectly defined but sessions should occur several times a week, with endurance time increasing gradually to at least 20 min or repetitions increasing to 30 with each task performed. Session duration and intensity can be monitored by the perceived severity of symptoms that occur. We do not monitor heart rate or oxyhaemoglobin saturation during arm exercise, although the heart rate is measured at the end of each session. Once the formal rehabilitation programme has been completed patients need to develop a self-directed exercise regimen to maintain any improvements which have occurred. Although this may not require the same frequency of training sessions, we encourage patients to perform their exercises daily in the hope that a routine will be developed and compliance enhanced.

Weight training

Weight training is an excellent method for improving upper-extremity performance and seems to be more effective than arm cycle ergometry. With legs, weight training also has a role, even though cycle ergometry is effective at improving leg performance. We recommend using weights for legs (in addition to cycling) in several groups of patients. In particular, weights can be applied for those who after a prolonged period of hospitalization or inactivity are too weak for cycle ergometry or for those whose pulmonary impairment makes meeting the ventilatory demands of general exercise too demanding. We also use weight training in patients in our rehabilitation programme who have well-preserved peripheral muscle function. In this group, who are usually younger than the average or with better lung function, we use weights in addition to a cycle and walking regimen.

Summary

Chronic airflow limitation leads to disability because of breathlessness. Deconditioning due to the reduction in activity, and other features of the condition such as malnourishment, aggravate the disability. Exercise training by improving peripheral muscle function is of benefit in decreasing the disability and resultant handicap, thereby improving quality of life. This section has aimed to show that isolated muscle group training, including weight-lifting exercises and specific upper-extremity exercise, should be an integral part of the treatment of these patients. Nevertheless, many questions still need to be answered.

Only the study of weight training by Simpson *et al.* (1992) assessed female patients with chronic airflow limitation and one wonders if the results in men can be generalized to the usual population seen in respiratory rehabilitation programmes. There is a need to determine the most effective and cost-effective training programme and to develop methods to enhance long-term compliance. The studies cited assessed exercise with upper extremities and the ventilatory response to the arm activity. The effect of training on the specific tasks of daily living which the patient finds troublesome has not been addressed. Do task performance, symptoms during specific tasks and quality of life improve? Hopefully the increasing interest in the mechanisms of benefit as a result of respiratory rehabilitation will lead to answers which will improve the treatment available to this group of individuals.

References

Allard, C., Jones, N.L., and Killian, K.J. (1989) Static peripheral skeletal muscle strength and exercise capacity in patients with chronic airflow limitation. *Am. Rev. Respir. Dis.* **139**:A90.

Belman, M.J., and Kendregan, B.A. (1981) Exercise training fails to increase skeletal muscle enzymes in patients with chronic obstructive pulmonary disease. *Am. Rev. Respir. Dis.* **123**:256–61.

Celli, B.R., Rassulo, J., and Make, B.J. (1986) Dyssynchronized breathing during arm but not leg exercise in patients with chronic airflow obstruction. *N. Engl. J. Med.* **314**:1485–90.

Couser, J.I., Martinez, F.J., and Celli, B.R. (1993) Pulmonary rehabilitation that includes arm exercise reduces metabolic and ventilatory requirements for simple arm elevation. *Chest* **103**:37–41.

Dolmage, T.E., Maestro, L., Avendano, M.A., and Goldstein, R.S. (1993) The ventilatory response to arm elevation of patients with chronic obstructive pulmonary disease. *Chest* **104**:1097–1100.

Guyatt, G., Berman, L.B., Townsend, M. *et al.* (1987) A measure of quality of life for clinical trials in chronic lung disease. *Thorax* **42**:773–8.

Lake, F.R., Henderson, K., Briffa, T. *et al.* (1990) Upper-limb and lower-limb exercise training in patients with chronic airflow obstruction. *Chest* **97**:1077–82.

Maltais, F., Simard, A.-A., Simard, L. *et al.* (1996) Oxidative capacity of the skeletal muscle and lactic acid kinetics during exercise in normal subjects and in patients with COPD. *Am. J. Respir. Crit. Care Med.* **153**:288–93.

Martinez, F.J., Couser, J.I., and Celli, B.R. (1991) Respiratory response to arm elevation in patients with chronic airflow limitation. *Am. Rev. Respir. Dis.* **143**:476–80.

Martinez, F.J., Vogel, P.D., Dupont, D.N. *et al.* (1993) Supported arm exercises vs unsupported arm exercise in the rehabilitation of patients with chronic airflow obstruction. *Chest* **103**:1397–1402.

Ries, A.L., Ellis, B., Hawkins, R.W. (1988) Upper extremity exercise training in chronic obstructive pulmonary disease. *Chest* **93**:688–92.

Simpson, K., Killian, K., McCartney, N. *et al.* (1992) Randomized control trial of weightlifting exercise in patients with chronic airflow limitation. *Thorax* **47**:70–5.

5. Nutrition – theoretical background and practical advice

J. Congleton

Chelsea and Westminster Hospital, London

Practical Pulmonary Rehabilitation.
Edited by Mike Morgan and Sally Singh.
Published in 1997 by Chapman & Hall, London.
ISBN 0 412 61810 9.

Introduction

Just as athletes pay attention to nutrition in order to optimize the performance of their body, so attention to nutrition is important for patients with chronic lung disease attending a rehabilitation programme. There are many reasons why nutrition may not be optimal in a patient with chronic obstructive pulmonary disease (COPD). COPD is more common in socioeconomic groups and geographical regions where diet is traditionally poor in terms of having a higher than average contribution from fat and a lower than average contribution from fresh vegetables and fruit. A low-activity lifestyle imposed by the disease may contribute to both obesity and skeletal muscle wasting. There may be problems in preparing meals if the kitchen is not suited to a person's disability and if there is difficulty in obtaining groceries due to restricted access to shopping facilities. In addition, some medications may affect food intake by causing gastrointestinal upset and corticosteroids may affect skeletal muscle synthesis, appetite and fat distribution.

The three common nutritional problems in pulmonary rehabilitation are malnutrition, obesity and diabetes mellitus. Malnutrition in COPD is not well understood scientifically and the standard techniques for dealing with it are not generally applicable to the COPD patient. For this reason there will be relatively greater emphasis on malnutrition in this text. Obesity is a common problem, as it is in the general population, and has the same underlying cause and management; however, these are compounded by respiratory restriction of activity and by oral corticosteroid medication. Diabetes mellitus is estimated to be present in between 1 and 2% of the general population. Prevalence increases with age, with obesity and can be induced by corticosteroids. Therefore diabetes commonly coexists with obesity in COPD patients and is managed as in the non-COPD patient. As a very rough estimate, in an average rehabilitation group 25–35% will be significantly underweight, 20–25% will be significantly overweight and 2% are likely to have non-insulin-dependent (type 2) diabetes mellitus.

In this chapter I aim to discuss current thinking on malnutrition in COPD. I will cover techniques of assessment of nutritional status and suggest ways of managing malnutrition and obesity in COPD.

Malnutrition in the COPD patient

Malnutrition and muscle wasting occur in a substantial proportion of patients with COPD with a number developing clinical protein-energy malnutrition. Unlike malnutrition caused by starvation, the cause is not well understood and the malnutrition is difficult to reverse. Its importance is that malnutrition in COPD has a direct effect on mortality as well as causing distress and malaise.

Impact of malnutrition in COPD

About a quarter to a third of outpatients with moderate to severe COPD are significantly underweight, with body weight less than 90% ideal (Muers and Green, 1993). Weight loss can progress at around 5–10% per year and then is a very difficult clinical problem as it is resistant to reversal despite active interventions. This type of malnutrition is protein-energy malnutrition (marasmus type) – there is loss of subcutaneous fat, severe muscle wasting, serum albumin is near normal, and there is no oedema. There is generally no evidence of micronutrient deficiency (vitamins and trace elements). Initially fat mass is lost and later both fat mass and fat-free mass become depleted. This is manifest initially by decrease in skinfold thickness, reflecting loss of fat, and later by both decrease in mid-arm circumference, reflecting loss of muscle, and clinically apparent muscle wasting. At its extreme, weight loss and muscle wasting can be dramatic and lead to concern that malignant disease is present, though there is only very occasionally an alternative explanation. Previously weight loss has been considered to be a problem limited to patients with emphysema as the prime diagnosis but in fact weight loss and muscle wasting can occur in any patient with COPD, whatever the prime pathophysiological diagnosis, though muscle wasting may be less apparent initially in a patient with cor pulmonale and fluid retention. The occurrence of weight loss cannot be predicted from any physiological variable, though there is some association with hypoxaemia.

Low weight in COPD is important as it is associated with increased mortality independent of respiratory function parameters (Wilson et al., 1989). In addition, muscle wasting may be very marked and reduced muscle mass leads to impairment of exercise performance. Muscle is made up of two fibre types: slow-twitch type 1 fibres and fast-twitch type 2 fibres. The effect of undernutrition on type 2 fibres is greater than that on type 1 fibres. The preferential atrophy of type 2 fibres has been suggested as the explanation for the observation of a stronger correlation between body weight and maximum oxygen consumption than that between body weight and endurance tests, as the strength during basal activities may be preserved but maximum power output will be impaired.

In common with cancer cachexia and muscular dystrophy, the mode of muscle depletion is by a reduction of muscle synthesis rather than increased muscle breakdown. The cause of this is not known for certain. Although the clinical picture is similar to that seen when energy intake is limited due to food shortage, decreased food intake does not appear to be the initiating factor. It has been suggested that cellular hypoxia is the cause of depressed muscle synthesis; however, muscle wasting is often most dramatic in the normoxaemic 'pink puffer'. A strong correlation between partial pressure of oxygen and muscle wasting has not been found, though it would seem more appropriate to examine whether there was a relation between muscle wasting and oxygen delivery to the tissues. Another possible explanation is that chronic malnutrition itself may contribute to depressed synthesis. Immobility leading to disuse atrophy may exacerbate muscle depletion. Corticosteroids also depress protein synthesis but severe wasting occurs just as commonly in patients who are not taking oral corticosteroids.

Potentially, effects on the respiratory muscles could be of great importance, as respiratory muscle fatigue and weakness could predispose to respiratory failure. The diaphragm is the main inspiratory muscle and postmortem studies in emphysema have found that diaphragm weight is lower than expected for body weight. A possible explanation for this is that respiratory muscle consists of a higher proportion of type 2 fibres than peripheral skeletal muscle and is therefore more susceptible to malnutrition than other muscles. Severe malnutrition can greatly reduce respiratory muscle strength in patients with no respiratory disease; however, there are conflicting reports of whether or not this is the case in malnourished COPD patients.

An increased susceptibility to certain types of infection due to decreased cell-mediated immunity is a feature of starvation-related malnutrition. This could potentially be important in COPD where a relatively minor infection could cause serious deterioration in status. However, tests of cell-mediated immunity (e.g. skin prick tests, total lymphocyte count) appear to be significantly abnormal only in COPD patients with extreme malnutrition and an increased incidence of infections in underweight patients has not been shown. Low body weight may be a factor in the lethargy and exhaustion that patients feel and there appears to be an independent relation between indices of malnutrition and quality of life (Congleton and Muers, 1995).

In summary, weight loss in COPD is associated with increased mortality independent of other factors and muscle wasting possibly contributes to respiratory muscle weakness.

Energy balance in malnourished COPD patients

For weight loss to occur, energy expenditure must exceed energy intake – there must be a state of negative energy balance. Negative energy balance occurs during exacerbations of COPD due to increased energy requirement related to illness and decreased food intake, and weight loss can occur over the period of a hospital stay. Recurrent exacerbations

---

Causes of negative energy balance

Reduced food intake

Reduced absorption of food

Increased energy expenditure

These may occur in isolation or in combination

Box 5.1

could therefore cause a stepwise weight loss. However, weight is usually regained if a full recovery is made, and the steady chronic loss which occurs despite a stable clinical state is probably more important for most patients. For an average-sized person a negative energy balance of 500 kJ/day would cause weight loss of 10% in about 1–2 years. Several of the medications commonly prescribed in COPD could theoretically contribute (theophylline can stimulate metabolism and salbutamol increases metabolic rate in the short term and can also decrease appetite) but the development of malnutrition does not appear to be related to medication.

Contribution of reduced energy intake and negative energy balance

Reduced food intake was initially assumed to be an important factor as there are many reasons why food intake could be reduced. For example, increased dyspnoea could limit intake due to irregular breathing while eating and swallowing, or due to increased gastric filling reducing functional residual capacity. It has also been suggested that patients with COPD may eat suboptimally because chewing and swallowing alter breathing pattern, which leads to arterial oxygen desaturation. This does not seem to occur in the majority of patients, though meal-related oxygen desaturation may be important in limiting intake in some hypoxic patients (Schols *et al.*, 1991a). Interpretation of food intake studies is difficult as dietary intake is notoriously difficult to assess; however, the present evidence implies that decreased food intake is not the *primary* cause of weight loss. Despite this, intake cannot be matching requirements if weight loss is occurring, and at some stage in the process difficulty increasing food intake sufficiently to match requirements must occur and thus exacerbate the situation.

Contribution of reduced absorption to negative energy balance

Malabsorption does not seem to be an important factor. No vitamin deficiencies were found in 27 COPD patients in one study and Semple *et al.*

Total energy expenditure in humans is the sum of three parts

Resting energy expenditure (REE; ≡ basal metabolic rate) – the energy expended by the body in its resting state, i.e. that required to keep the organs 'ticking over'

Diet-induced thermogenesis (DIT) – the energy expenditure associated with processing and storing food

Exercise-induced energy expenditure – the energy expended due to any activity over and above the resting state

Box 5.2

(1979) carried out detailed malabsorption studies on 8 severely underweight COPD patients including jejunal biopsy, faecal fat estimation, *d*-xylose excretion, iron, vitamin B_{12} and folate estimation and found normal results in all.

Contribution of increased energy expenditure to negative energy balance

Total energy expenditure in humans is the sum of resting energy expenditure (REE), diet-induced energy expenditure and the energy expended by activity. By far the greatest component is REE, which accounts for 60–80% of total energy expenditure in normal subjects. It varies with age, sex and the amount of metabolically active tissue, of which fat-free mass gives an estimate. Diet-induced thermogenesis accounts for around 15% of total energy expenditure and the energy expended by activity is a small fraction of the total. Patients with respiratory disease have a greater oxygen cost for a given level of activity but this is offset by their reduced level of activity and therefore is not felt to be the cause of their negative energy balance. Feeding studies examining whether there is an increase in diet-induced thermogenesis give conflicting results. It is possible that diet-induced thermogenesis may be increased in COPD compared to normal subjects but if this is the case, it is not to a great degree.

An elevation of REE by 10–20% would be sufficient to cause the degree of weight loss observed. REE can be measured by indirect calorimetry and is found to be elevated by this amount in a proportion of COPD patients. This is a particularly important observation as the physiological response to semistarvation is for REE to fall. This therefore supports the view that undereating is not the *primary* cause of weight loss in these patients, as it would be expected to be associated with a low REE.

The hypothesis that an elevation of REE is the cause of weight loss is an attractive proposition and has received much support. It has been suggested that this is in turn caused by the increased work of breathing, though this is hard to prove as work of breathing is difficult to measure in the true resting state. However, elevation of REE occurs in some weight-stable patients and conversely REE may be normal in weight-losing COPD patients. In addition, a study of total 24-h energy expenditure in COPD showed no increase in total daily energy expenditure compared to control subjects, i.e. the increased energy expenditure due to elevation of REE in the COPD patients was totally offset by a spontaneous reduction in activity (Hugli *et al.*, 1996).

The clinical appearance of malnourished COPD patients is very similar to that in cardiac cachexia, chronic liver disease and malignancy, which suggests that there may be a systemic cause. Tumour necrosis factor, a cytokine, has been noted to be raised in hypermetabolic COPD patients. Although this is a non-specific marker, it again supports a systemic cause and more work in this area is awaited.

Reversing malnutrition in COPD – is it possible?

Unlike other weight-losing patients, e.g. those with severe burns or septic patients, COPD patients are not catabolic – they do not exhibit a greater nitrogen breakdown than expected for a given energy expenditure. This means that, in theory, calorie supplementation will lead to weight gain (Goldstein *et al.*, 1988). Disappointingly, this has been extremely difficult to achieve in practice. Controlled studies of refeeding underweight COPD patients have given generally poor results (Fitting, 1992). A high calorie intake is required to show weight gain, for example 1.7 times measured REE, and this amount is often difficult for patients to achieve with oral supplementation alone. Weight gain that has been achieved has been small and not maintained. Any improvement in respiratory muscle strength, walking distance or other functional parameters has also been small but has seemed to occur in tandem with weight gain. Once the patients are no longer encouraged to continue their diets there is a spontaneous rapid reduction of intake back to preintervention levels and a slower fall in weight and physiological measures back to pretreatment levels over several months. In addition, some recent work shows that any increase in weight appears to be solely due to increase of fat mass without increase in fat-free mass (Donahoe *et al.*, 1994).

Varying the type of feed does not seem to lead to a great difference in results. As the exercise capacity of most COPD patients is limited primarily by ventilation, a large carbohydrate load could theoretically overload the respiratory system as carbohydrate leads to increase in carbon dioxide production compared to fat with the same calorific value. High carbohydrate feeds have been reported to contribute to difficulty weaning from a ventilator. This effect does not seem to be important in the stable state and there have been no reports of worsening respiratory failure attributed to carbohydrate loads in this situation. One study showed that a fat-based drink led to reduced increase in partial pressure of carbon dioxide, minute ventilation and less decrease in 6 min walking distance 30 min after feeding than a carbohydrate-based drink (Efthimiou *et al.*, 1993). However, the differences involved were small and it is not clear whether the differences are clinically important.

It seems likely that refeeding alone is not an effective treatment for the majority of undernourished COPD patients and an additional or alternative approach will be necessary to give good results. The general lack of success highlights the importance of the need for further research into the mechanism of weight loss as this may lead to development of effective interventions. Current strategies under investigation are the use of growth hormone, anabolic steroids and muscle training, all in conjunction with ensuring adequate calorie intake.

Whatever the cause of weight loss and a hypermetabolic state in COPD, the practical implications are that patients should be monitored for signs of early malnutrition as we are much more likely to be able to manage the problem if it is detected early. Adequacy of nutrition should be assessed in all COPD patients with the aim of preventing malnutrition occurring. Any planned refeeding regimen should take account of the fact that energy requirements are likely to be elevated by at least 20% of expected. In addition, there will be an even higher calorie requirement to normal when patients are taking part in a rehabilitation programme due to increased physical activity.

Nutritional assessment of patients in a pulmonary rehabilitation programme

Use of body weight in assessment

Both present weight and indication of weight change are important. More meaning is given to present weight by expressing it taking other parameters into account. A common method is to express weight as a percentage of the ideal body weight (%IBW). The IBW depends on height, bone frame and age, and can be obtained from tables or from prediction formulae (Blaque-Belair *et al.*, 1980; Metropolitan Life Insurance Company, 1983). For patients with COPD, a weight less than 90% IBW should be considered significantly low. Another widely used measure is the body mass index (BMI), which is equivalent to weight in kilograms

---

Parameters used in assessing nutritional status

Body weight

Body mass index

% Ideal body weight

Fat mass

Fat-free mass

Visceral protein status

Box 5.3

Equations for calculation of % ideal body weight (IBW) and body mass index (BMI)

$$\%\text{IBW} = \frac{\text{Actual weight (kg)}}{\left[\left(\text{height(in cm)} - 100\right) + \left(\text{age}/10\right)\right] \times 0.9} \times 100\%$$

Or obtain IBW from tables, e.g. Metropolitan Life Insurance Tables (1983)

$$\text{BMI} = \text{weight(in kg)}/\text{height}^2(\text{in m}) \quad \text{kg/m}^2$$

Box 5.4

---

divided by the square of the height in metres. Equations for calculating %IBW and BMI are given in Box 5.4.

A guide to the values of %IBW and BMI is given in Table 5.1 and recognized grades of malnutrition and obesity are given in Tables 5.2 and 5.3.

Change in weight from previous weight is more difficult to assess, though it can sometimes be obtained from the case records. However, patients usually present after becoming unwell and therefore there is often no record of their normal weight. Many patients accurately remember their previous steady weight ('I was 11 stone 8 on the day I got married and I weighed exactly the same on my 40th birthday'), though this good recall is not the case in all. When monitoring serial weight it is important to weigh the patient on each occasion under standard conditions, e.g. shoeless in light clothing on the same scales (or to be sure that different sets of scales give comparable readings by calibrating them with known weights). A loss of 5% of body weight over a year is generally taken as significant loss.

Table 5.1 Guide to equivalent values of % ideal body weight (IBW) and body mass index (BMI)

%IBM	BMI	Nutritional status
<70%	<16 kg/m^2	Severe malnutrition
71%–80%	16–18.4 kg/m^2	Moderate malnutrition
80%–90%	18.5–20.9 kg/m^2	At risk
90%–110%	21–24.9 kg/m^2	Desirable
110%–120%	25–29.9 kg/m^2	Moderate obesity
>120%	>30 kg/m^2	Severe obesity

Note that these measures are not strictly comparable; the groupings are meant to give a rough guide of equivalents.

Also note that both IBW and BMI reflect the present state and give no indication of how weight has changed over time.

Table 5.2 The international dietary energy consultancy group grades of malnutrition

Body mass index	Grade of malnutrition
<18.5 kg/m^2	Grade I
<17 kg/m^2	Grade II
<16 kg/m^2	Grade III

Table 5.3 Grading of obesity

Body mass index	Grade of obesity
25–29.9 kg/m^2	Grade I
30–39.9 kg/m^2	Grade II
>40 kg/m^2	Grade III

From Garrow and Webster (1985), with permission.

Use of body composition in assessment

More information about nutritional status can be obtained by assessing body composition, or the relative proportions of the body's components. Assessment of all the different body constituents in a live being would be very complex, and impractical in clinical practice and those that we are most interested in are muscle, fat and water. A simple way of considering body composition is to divide the body into two compartments – fat mass and fat-free mass (Fig. 5.1). (Fat-free mass can also be called lean body mass.) Fat mass consists of adipose tissue. Fat-free mass consists largely of muscle but also contains bone and the major visceral organs. Muscle accounts for approximately 50% of the fat-free mass. Water is not present in fat, it is only distributed in the fat-free mass and normally accounts for 73% of this by weight. Even in cor pulmonale it seems that the total amount of water is unchanged but that it is distributed differently in the body. It follows that if we can measure one of these components – fat mass, fat-free mass or total body water – and know the body weight, we can deduce the others, as shown in Box 5.5.

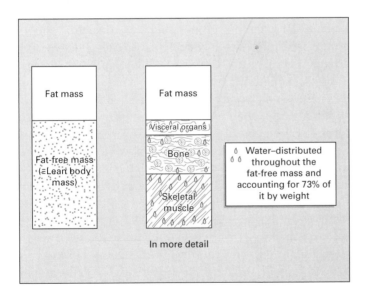

Fig. 5.1 The two-compartment model of body composition.

Calculating fat mass (FM), fat-free mass (FFM) and total body water (TBW)

Body weight = FFM + FM

$0.73 \times \text{FFM} = \text{TBW}$

Box 5.5   137

The value of the constituents can be expressed as an absolute value in kilograms or as a percentage of the body weight. But it must be remembered that an apparent increase in the percentage of one component (e.g. fat-free mass) could be entirely accounted for by a decrease in another (e.g. fat mass). In addition, values need interpreting in the context of body weight. Thus, percentage values can be useful for comparison of groups of subjects but for serial measurement of one patient it is probably preferable to monitor absolute values. It is reasonable to assume that the weight of visceral organs and skeleton does not change much, and then fat-free mass gives an indication of muscle mass. The prime aim of nutritional intervention is to maintain or replete fat-free mass.

Normal body composition differs for men and women; the main difference is that the normal state is for women to have relatively more fat. An important point is that there is a physiological change in body composition with increasing age. Fat-free mass declines between the ages of 20 and 70 years, from an average of 60 kg to 50 kg in men, and from an average of 40 kg to 35 kg in women, i.e. at a rate of 200 g per year. Muscle mass falls from 450 g/kg body weight to 300 g/kg body weight. Over a similar time scale the percentage body fat rises from 20% to 30% in men and from 27% to 40% in women. In addition, in the elderly a redistribution of fat occurs, from peripheral areas such as the arms and legs, to central areas such as the abdomen. The change in the above variables with age highlights the importance of comparing patients' values to age- and sex-related standards; and when planning clinical studies the importance of obtaining control subjects matched for age and sex.

The measurement of body composition can give an indication of nutritional status, as faced with nutritional restriction the body utilizes reserves stored mainly as skeletal protein, visceral protein and fat. Change in skeletal protein is indicated by changes in fat-free mass or muscle mass, and change in fat stores is indicated by fat mass. It is therefore also possible to detect muscle wasting which is being masked by an increase in body fat. In addition, the status of visceral protein stores is indicated by serum levels of certain proteins synthesized by the body (albumin, prealbumin, transferrin and retinol-binding protein). However, these proteins are negative acute-phase proteins and therefore can be falsely low if measured in the acute inflammatory state.

There are many possible ways of assessing body composition but in clinical practice suitable methods are skinfold anthropometry and bio-electrical impedance. Other methods, such as densitometry, dilution of radioactively labelled water and absorptiometry, require expensive equipment and resources and are more applicable to a basic research setting. However, dual-energy X-ray absorptiometry is used increasingly to assess bone density in clinical practice and the weight of fat mass and

Methods of measuring body composition

Anthropometry, using skinfold thickness

Bioelectrical impedance (BIA)

Dual-energy X-ray absorptiometry (DEXA)

Underwater weighing

Dilution of heavy water

Total body potassium

Creatinine height index

Box 5.6

To measure skinfold thickness

■ Grasp the skin and subcutaneous tissue at the correct site (Fig. 5.2), between the thumb and forefinger of the left hand (assuming the recorder is right-handed)

■ Shake the tissue gently to exclude underlying muscle

■ Pull the tissue at right angles away from the body just enough to allow application of the calliper jaws

■ Allow the calliper jaws to close by releasing the handle

■ The needle on the dial will fall quickly initially, then slowly for a few seconds and the reading should be taken at the end of this second period as soon as the needle has come to a rest

■ It is best to take three readings at each site and, providing they agree reasonably well, take the average of the three readings as the skinfold thickness at that site

Box 5.7

fat-free mass can be obtained from the results of the same scan. Creatinine height index, although cheap and apparently simple to perform, is not recommended for clinical assessment as it can produce variable results and there are many possible errors in the technique. Comprehensive reviews of the various methods for assessing body composition are given by Lukaski (1987) and Burkinshaw (1985).

Practical use of skinfold anthropometry

Fat mass can be estimated from subcutaneous fat by measurement of skinfold thicknesses using skinfold callipers which are designed so that the jaws exert a constant pressure of $10 \, g/mm^2$ of contact area. One

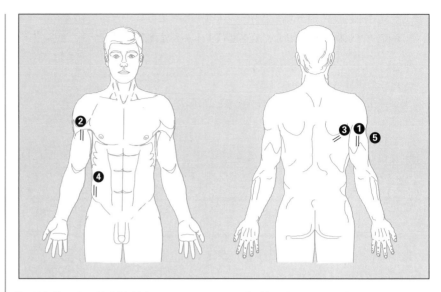

Fig. 5.2 Sites for skinfold thickness measurements. Position the arm with the elbow flexed at a right angle to feel the bony landmarks and, using a tape measure, make a pen mark at the mid-point of the upper arm over the triceps belly.

1. *Triceps* – over the triceps muscle halfway between the tip of the acromion at the shoulder and the olecranon at the elbow, parallel to the long axis of the arm. The arm should be hanging relaxed by the side of the body.
2. *Biceps* – over the mid-point of the muscle belly at the same point as the triceps skinfold on the opposite side of the arm parallel to the long axis of the arm. Again, the arm should be hanging relaxed by the side of the body.
3. *Subscapular* – 1–2 cm below the tip of the inferior angle of the scapula at an angle of 45° to the vertical.
4. *Suprailiac* – Just above the iliac crest in the mid-axillary line, parallel with the long axis of the body.
5. *Mid-arm circumference (MAC)* – measured with a tape measure at the mid-point between the acromion and the olecranon process with the arm hanging relaxed at the side.

model of callipers is made by British Indicators Ltd (Burgess Hill, UK) and is available in analogue and digital versions; personally, I have found the analogue version easier to use. The method for measurement is described in Box 5.7 and the sites for measurement in Figure 5.2.

The ease of measurement varies with the subject's fatness and the consistency of the subcutaneous tissue. The accuracy of the technique depends on the operator's skill; however, reproducibility improves with practice. It is worth gaining expertise on all available willing subjects and formally recording the reproducibility of the technique in your hands before commencing measurements on patients. Advantages of this method are that it is cheap, quick and the equipment is easily portable.

The results from skinfold thicknesses can be used in various ways:

1. Using four-site skinfold thickness to estimate fat mass.
2. Using triceps skinfold and mid-arm muscle circumference to indicate fat and protein stores.
3. Using arm fat area and arm muscle area to indicate fat and protein stores.
4. Using serial change of any index.

USING FOUR-SITE SKINFOLD THICKNESS TO ESTIMATE FAT MASS

Skinfold thickness is measured at four sites: triceps, biceps, subscapular and suprailiac. The measurements are made on one side of the body, usually the right side, though the side used does not seem to be important. The skinfold thicknesses at each of these four sites are added together and this value can be used to estimate fat mass with the equations or tables of Durnin and Wormersley (1974). The appropriate equation depends on the age and gender of the subject. Alternatively, fewer than four skinfolds can be measured; for example, it may be decided that it is more convenient to measure triceps and biceps only. Durnin and Wormersley's paper gives equations for the derivation of fat mass for any combination of the skinfolds but, as the method assumes that the thickness of the subcutaneous adipose tissue reflects a constant proportion of body fat and that the sites selected for measurement are representative of subcutaneous adipose tissue, a more accurate result is obtained if more sites are selected. The method compares well with more sophisticated methods and has been validated in COPD patients (Schols *et al.*, 1991b).

USING TRICEPS SKINFOLD AND MID-ARM MUSCLE CIRCUMFERENCE TO
INDICATE FAT AND PROTEIN STORES

Another way of using anthropometry is to use triceps skinfold (TSF) thickness and mid-arm muscle circumference to indicate nutritional status. Mid-arm circumference (MAC) is measured in the non-dominant arm with a cloth tape-measure. The measurement is made at the mid-point between the acromion and olecranon and the mean of three readings is taken as MAC. Mid-arm muscle circumference (MAMC) can be calculated from TSF and MAC by assuming that the arm is roughly circular in cross-section.

MAMC is taken to reflect stores of skeletal protein and triceps skinfold is an indicator of calorie reserves stored as fat. Together they can be used as an indicator of protein-energy malnutrition by comparing the values to normal percentiles (Frisancho, 1981). For example, if a patient has both TSF and MAMC lying on the 50th centile, that person has average fat and skeletal protein stores. If a patient has measurements of TSF on the 5th centile and MAMC lying between the 25th and 50th centile, this would indicate that there is loss of fat stores with relative preservation of skeletal protein stores; this is the normal initial response

Box 5.8

Calculation of mid-arm muscle circumference (MAMC)

$$\text{MAMC} = \text{MAC} - \left(\pi \times \text{TSF} \right)$$

MAC = Mid-arm circumference; TSF = triceps skinfold thickness; $\pi \approx 3.14$.

Calculating arm muscle area (AMA) and arm fat area (AFA)

Males $\qquad \text{AMA} = \left[\dfrac{\left(\text{MAC} - \pi\text{TSF} \right)^2}{4\pi} \right] - 10$

Females $\qquad \text{AMA} = \left[\dfrac{\left(\text{MAC} - \pi\text{TSF} \right)^2}{4\pi} \right] - 6.5$

Males + females $\qquad \text{AFA} = \dfrac{\text{MAC}^2}{4\pi} - \text{AMA}$

MAC = mid-arm circumference; TSF = triceps skinfold thickness.

Alternatively, AMA and AFA can be obtained from TSF and MAC using published nomograms (Gurney and Jellife, 1973).

Box 5.9

to starvation. However, a patient whose TSF lies between the 25th and 50th centile and AMC on the 5th centile has some loss of fat stores but extreme skeletal protein depletion.

USING ARM FAT AREA AND ARM MUSCLE AREA TO INDICATE FAT AND PROTEIN STORES

The cross-sectional areas of both arm muscle and arm fat are probably better indications of nutritional status than TSF and MAMC because these measures can both underestimate the tissue changes that can occur in the upper arm when nutritional status changes. Arm fat area and arm muscle area can both be worked out from TSF and MAC. Allowing for the fact that the arm is not an exact cylinder and that the bone shape is irregular, the equations according to Heymsfield *et al.* (1982) are given in Box 5.9. As before, an assessment of nutritional status is made by comparison to published norms (Frisancho, 1981).

USING SERIAL CHANGE OF ANY INDEX

This is perhaps most useful for follow-up of patients once their nutritional status has been assessed and documented. A word of caution is not to overinterpret changes that may be due to the normal variation of the technique. Serial change in body weight could be usefully tracked monthly; however, an interval of 2–3 months is recommended for tracking changes in body composition due to the inherent variability of measurements.

Practical use of bioelectrical impedance

This is a relatively new technique which is being used increasingly. Impedance of the flow of a small electrical current applied at the skin surface is measured with a specifically designed meter. The method uses the difference between the good conduction of ions in body fluids as opposed to the poor conductivity of fat to give an estimate of total body water, from which the amount of fat-free mass can be derived. The reading is very simple and quick to perform, painless and safe and the machinery is relatively inexpensive (≈£500) and easily portable. The technique is much less susceptible to inter- and intraobserver error than the measurement of skinfold thickness. It has been validated as a reliable method in stable COPD patients (Schols *et al.*, 1991b), though the effect of changes of body water distribution, for example in cor pulmonale, on the measurement is not known. One problem is that the impedance reading alone means little and an absurd reading, for example one that

---

Summary of information from anthropometry and bioelectrical impedance

- FM (and therefore FFM) from the sum of 4 (or less) skinfold thicknesses
- Percentile of TSF and MAC to indicate loss of fat stores and protein stores respectively
- Percentile of AFA and AMA to indicate fat stores and protein stores respectively
- FM (and therefore FFM) from bioelectrical impedance

FM = Fat mass; FFM = fat-free mass; TSF = triceps skinfold thickness; MAC = mid-arm circumference; AFA = arm fat area; AMA = arm muscle area

Box 5.10

gives a body water weight greater than the total body weight, may not be recognized until the results are calculated at a later time, i.e. when the patient has gone home. Another problem is that the manufacturer's equations (often included in the machine software) may not be the best equations to use to convert impedance into total body water and ideally regression equations should be specifically generated for the COPD population by comparison to reference methods for assessing body composition for each make of machine. This has been done for the model made by RJL (Schols *et al.*, 1991b).

Visceral protein status

Visceral protein status can also be assessed by measurement of serum proteins such as transferrin and albumin; however, it is not recommended that these are measured routinely as serum protein levels are rarely low in COPD unless the degree of malnutrition is extreme (e.g. <70% IBW). In addition they may act as negative acute-phase proteins – levels may fall in the presence of inflammation.

Management of nutrition in a pulmonary rehabilitation programme (Box 5.11)

Input from a dietitian is invaluable in order to make a complete assessment. The first step is to document nutritional status and I would recommend that all patients entering a rehabilitation programme have their nutritional status assessed. The rehabilitation programme should have a standard assessment protocol so that the persons involved become familiar with the method of expressing body weight and composition that the team is using. I would recommend that some assessment of body composition is made if at all possible. I would not recommend the routine measurement of serum proteins for the reasons discussed.

The next step is to assess nutritional intake. A skilled dietitian is particularly important for this part as dietary histories are very difficult to take accurately. As malnutrition is difficult to reverse once marked weight loss has occurred, it seems logical to attempt to prevent it occurring by attention to food intake in all patients. In addition, a minor degree of obesity that would cause no harm to an otherwise healthy person may increase respiratory work in the COPD patient. A full assessment includes not only food intake but also meal patterns and problems related to food intake.

The two main methods used to assess food intake are 24-h recall and dietary history. Using these techniques and food reference tables the dietitian will be able to estimate energy intake and proportions of the

*Management of nutrition
in a pulmonary
rehabilitation programme*

Nutritional management of patients entering rehabilitation programme

Assessment – all patients
Nutritional status
Nutritional intake
Special nutritional needs
Patients with evidence of obesity
Clinical assessment, review steroid dose
Decide target weight
Education
Plan individual programme of reduced intake
Review, ? reached goal
Continue regular review
Patients with diabetes mellitus
Clinical assessment, review steroid dose
Review knowledge of diabetes
Plan altered diet/medication as appropriate
Review, ? improved control
Patients with evidence of malnutrition or early malnutrition
Clinical assessment
Plan nutritional support
Review, ? reached goal

Box 5.11

Recording nutritional status

Weight
An estimate of rate of weight loss or gain
Either % ideal body weight or body mass index
Some measure of fat and skeletal protein store (skinfolds or bioelectrical impedance)

Box 5.12

main constituents of diet (fat, carbohydrate and protein). Any physical problems affecting intake should be explored, such as ill-fitting dentures, loss of appetite and breathlessness during eating. Socioeconomic factors should also be considered, for example social isolation or boredom which may lead to behavioural overeating, problems preparing food in an unsuitable kitchen or difficulty getting out to buy shopping. Other factors which may be important should be considered, such as the presence of

Box 5.13

> ## Methods of assessment of dietary intake
>
> *24-h recall*
> Retrospective interview into food intake over the previous day
> Relatively simple and quick
> Assumes that intake is representative of the week
> Tends to underestimate intake as foods are easily forgotten
>
> *Dietary history*
> Retrospective interview to ascertain typical intake over past few weeks or months
> Establish a weekly pattern
> Can build in cross-checks, e.g. with amount of butter purchased over a time period
> Time-consuming
> Can use combination of the two, i.e. 24-h recall with reference to variations over the week
>
> *Food diary*
> 3-day food diary most commonly used
> Records amounts of all food eaten over 2 week-days and 1 weekend-day
> Needs a high degree of patient motivation

other diseases which may have their own dietary needs. Once problems are identified, these can be used to guide recommendations.

Clinical assessment

All patients with an identified nutritional problem should be assessed clinically with the problem in mind. Carry out a focused history and examination on one occasion. COPD patients have often been attending the clinic for many years and attention may not have been turned to other systems for some time. Investigations should be ordered as indicated from the clinical assessment, such as thyroid function tests, haemoglobin and faecal occult bloods, and sputum for acid- and alcohol-fast bacilli. The patient may not have had a chest X-ray for some time; if this is the case, one should be ordered, or if there is a relatively recent chest X-ray look at it on this occasion to observe for lesions suspicious of carcinoma or tuberculosis. Although there is usually no other cause found, many of the reported series of weight loss in COPD include a few patients in whom a previously unsuspected carcinoma was later diagnosed. Consider whether any medication may be contributing and alter drug therapy as appropriate. It is important to take an accurate drug history;

patients may be taking more steroids than realized: 'a few more when I feel a bit rough'. For most COPD patients it is possible to wean or reduce maintenance oral corticosteroids over time. This is particularly important for the overweight or diabetic patient. Therapy that may be causing indigestion should be reconsidered or indigestion treated. Optimizing medical management is obviously important; weight loss does occur in acute exacerbations and the patient will benefit from the nutritional point of view by these episodes being kept to a minimum. During an acute exacerbation attention should be paid to nutritional intake to attempt to minimize loss.

Managing the overweight COPD patient

The aim of management is to achieve weight loss and to maintain this weight in the future. The principles of achieving this are similar in anyone who is overweight and consist of attempting to change eating behaviour long term. In the general population intervention is indicated for grade II and III obesity but in the context of COPD it may be appropriate at grade I. A thorough assessment of overweight patients requires sensitivity and attention to detail. Food diaries tend to be particularly inaccurate in overweight patients and it is important to carry out cross-checks by assessing weekly shopping amounts and with the co-habitees. It is important to try and understand the person's eating habits and discover behavioural or psychological factors that have a bearing on these. It is also important to deal in the context of the people with whom they normally eat or who prepare their meals. It is important to discover if weight loss has been attempted previously and if so why these attempts failed.

After this assessment, a realistic target weight should be decided on, taking into account the patient's previous weight and how long the patient has been overweight. It may be advisable in addition to aim for a short-term achievable goal initially, e.g. 5 kg or 1 stone over 6 months. Even this amount of weight loss may have a significant impact on a person's well-being and if reached, will have a very positive effect on the patient's psyche. The next step is to educate and motivate the patient. It is extremely important to convey to the patient that weight *can* be lost by eating less in the way of calories. Many patients find this hard to believe and are convinced that their metabolism is slow and that they will never lose weight 'even if they eat nothing'. It is important to deal with the issue of oral steroids. Steroids do increase appetite and this can be satiated by eating foods with very low calorie content. In addition, steroids cause fat to be distributed centrally rather than peripherally so that the patient appears fatter.

The other aspect of education is related to the quality of the diet and the calorie content of differing foods in conjunction with advice on measures to cut calorie intake. An individual programme is devised for each patient. Protein intake needs to be maintained so that skeletal muscle is not lost, but this is not a problem for most people in the UK. The main aim is to reduce or substitute fat in diet and this is mainly achieved by changing to low-fat substitutes and altering cooking habits. An increase in fruit and vegetables is good for satiety and provides micronutrients. Regular lower-calorie meals are encouraged rather than missing meals as this is likely to provoke hunger and binges. A particular difficulty is that appetite may increase during the course of a programme with increased activity.

Weight change is likely to be slow and it must be explained that day-to-day variations are due to change in water or the scales. Motivation can be a problem; however, in the context of the rehabilitation programme, probably less so. The group atmosphere may provide additional motivation, support and encouragement but apparent 'failures' need to be dealt with sensitively. Arrange review to see if the target has been reached and if so, aim to maintain it.

Planning nutritional support in malnourished patients

To guide nutritional replacement one needs to make an estimate of energy expenditure. A few centres have access to indirect calorimetry to measure REE but this is primarily a research tool. The Harris–Benedict equation (Harris and Benedict, 1919) gives a close estimate of REE in normal subjects using age, sex, height and weight but, as discussed, it tends to underestimate the energy requirements of COPD patients. An alternative prediction equation is the Scholfield (1985) formula. As there is no way of predicting which patients have an elevated REE, in the absence of a measure of REE I would suggest assuming a REE of 1.2 times that predicted by the Harris–Benedict equation for all patients. From trials of refeeding in COPD, the energy intake required to achieve weight gain is 1.7 times the measured REE – this allows for exercise-related energy expenditure and diet-induced thermogenesis.

Although there are theoretical advantages of aiming for a relatively high fat intake in relation to reducing carbon dioxide excretion, there is no evidence to support strongly a particular ratio of fat to carbohydrate intake and the main aim is to achieve the target calorie intake. In addition, a proportion of patients find a diet high in fat difficult to cope with due to early satiety. The protein intake required for gain in fat-free mass is not known for certain but as these patients are not catabolic, protein intake should not need to be too high, providing calorie intake is sufficient. The reference nutrient intake (i.e. 2 s.d. above the estimated average requirement) for protein for adults in the UK is 0.75 g/kg per

---

Harris – Benedict equation

Male   Estimated REE = 66.4730 + 13.7516w
                             + 5.0033h − 6.7550a

Female   Estimated REE = 665.0955 + 9.5643w
                             + 1.8496h − 4.6756a

REE = Resting energy expenditure in 24 h (calories); w = weight in kg; h = height in cm; a = age in years.

Estimated energy requirements for nutritional repletion in chronic obstructive pulmonary disease = 1.7 × 1.2 × estimated REE.

Box 5.14

day, but in fact most people eat plenty of protein. The reference nutrient intake is only valid if energy intake is sufficient; otherwise protein is used as a source of energy rather than for synthesis. Using information from trials which have shown improvement in nutritional status in COPD, it has been suggested that a protein intake of 1.7 g/kg per day should be aimed for (Mancino *et al.*, 1993). When commencing nutritional support it is important to ensure that other related aspects are satisfactory; for example, that dentition is adequate and that any dentures are well-fitting, that there are mechanisms in place for getting the shopping, and that there is sufficient money and the intention to use it for food.

Once target intake has been decided upon, dietary counselling attempts to encourage the patient to increase oral food intake, e.g. by boosting nutrient-dense foods such as milk, butter and cream to reach these goals. Close monitoring by a dietitian is very important. The problems identified in the nutritional intake assessment should be addressed. For example, if anorexia is a problem, frequent high-calorie meals should be recommended. If breathlessness during eating is a problem, the patient may benefit from education on breathing control, advice to rest before a meal and to eat slowly. Soft, moist semisolid foods are generally easier to manage. If sufficient intake is achieved the patient should continue to receive dietary counselling as maintaining intake requires effort.

If food intake cannot be increased to reach the target intake, consider adding oral supplements. The important point is that these are, as their name suggests, a supplement and not a replacement for food. Therefore they should be taken at the end of the meal and in between meals so that food intake is not reduced. Before bed is a good time for supplements and guidance on their administration is essential. Some measure of body composition should be monitored if these are being instituted to

149

> ## Overview of techniques used in nutritional support in chronic obstructive pulmonary disease
>
> 1. Education
> 2. Increase oral intake
> 3. Oral supplements
> 4. Supplementary enteral nutrition: nasogastric/percutaneous endoscopic gastrostomy
>
> The approach is modelled on that used in cystic fibrosis which has been shown to lead to success. However, to date it seems that nutritional repletion is much harder to achieve in patients with chronic obstructive pulmonary disease. There is a stepwise use of techniques, nearly always starting at 1 and working up to 4 if necessary. Achievement of target should be regularly reviewed, including assessment of fat mass and fat-free mass.

Box 5.15

record change in both fat mass and fat-free mass. Again, increased intake will need to be sustained and follow-up and reinforcement of advice are important. Monitoring of nutritional status should continue on a 2–3-monthly basis.

If intake cannot be sufficiently increased with food and oral supplements, the next step to consider is supplementary enteral feeding. This can be administered via either a nasogastric tube or a gastrostomy. There are many advantages of a gastrostomy and this method has had very good results in patients with cystic fibrosis. The tube is relatively simple to place percutaneously and there are few complications. It is difficult to give guidelines for when this is appropriate as there is no strong supporting evidence of its success in COPD. However, if the patient is clearly unable to increase oral intake sufficiently to a reasonable level, then it should be considered with monitoring of nutritional status to assess response. It is helpful if the clinical team has pre-agreed criteria for initiating this intervention.

In conclusion, malnutrition is a debilitating condition and understanding of the cause is incomplete at present. Appropriate attention to nutritional status and nutritional intake may help prevent frank malnutrition developing. More effective techniques for nutritional intervention are needed; meanwhile, any planned intervention should take into account the increased energy expenditure that occurs in some patients. Overweight patients may believe that there is no way they can lose weight; however, the cause of weight gain is known and good results can be achieved with due care to education and motivation, though it can be hard to achieve. The results of nutritional intervention should be monitored by appropriate techniques, including an assessment of fat and protein stores.

Appendix 5A

S. Pitten and S. Patel

Treating poor appetite and weight loss

The first line of approach in improving or preventing deterioration in a patient's nutritional status is to encourage the patient to increase the amount of oral diet taken and ensure that meals are well balanced. This can be achieved by taking larger or more frequent meals and snacks. However, it is important that the patient is advised regarding the appropriate consistency and texture of meals.

When sufficient quantities and a normal diet are managed, patients should be encouraged to fortify their meals – fortification of the diet is a method employed to improve the energy and protein content of the diet.

Practical suggestions

Increase the use of dairy products:

■ Add grated cheese, milk powder or cream to soups and sauces (choose full-fat varieties).
■ Add extra butter or margarine and/or milk to mashed potato and vegetables.
■ Grate cheese into mashed potato.

Foods should be included from the following groups daily:

■ **Protein**, e.g. meat, poultry, fish, dairy products, beans, lentils, dhal and nuts.
■ **Starchy foods**, e.g. bread, other cereals and potatoes.
■ **Fruit and vegetables**, e.g. fresh, frozen, pure fruit juice.
■ **Dairy products**, e.g. milk, cheese, yoghurts, fromage frais – ensure full-fat varieties are chosen.

■ Fry foods rather than grilling.
■ Use jam, syrup and treacle in recipes. Add sugar or glucose to drinks and desserts.
■ Milk can be fortified – to half a litre of milk add 4 tablespoons of milk

powder, e.g. Five Pints or Marvel. Use this for porridge, cereals, milk drinks, milk puddings, soups and sauces.

■ Drink fluids after meals.

■ Make use of convenience foods which require very little preparation.

■ If unable to manage a full meal, try a milkshake or supplemental soup and pudding as an alternative.

Prescribable supplements	*Non-prescribable supplements*
Fortisip	Complan
Fresubin	Build-up
Ensure Plus	Build-up soup
Provide	Vita food
Maxijul powder	
Maxijul liquid	
Enlive	
Hycal	
(This is not a complete list)	

All need to be administered under medical/dietetic supervision.

References

Blaque-Belair, A., deFossey, B., and Restier, M. (1980) *Dictionnaire des constantes biologique et physiologiques*. Paris: Maloire, p. 1648.

Burkinshaw, L. (1985) Measurement of human body composition *in vivo*. In: *Progress in Medical Radiation Physics*, Vol. 2 (ed. C.G. Orton). London: Plenum, pp. 113–37.

Congleton, J., and Muers, M.F. (1995) Relation of nutritional indices to quality of life in COPD. *Eur. Respir. J.* **8** (suppl. 19):172s (abstract).

Donahoe, M., Mancino, J., Costantino, J. *et al.* (1994) The effect of an aggressive nutritional support regimen on body composition in patients with severe COPD and weight loss. *Am. Rev. Respir. Dis.* **A313** (abstract).

Durnin, J.V.G.A., and Wormersley, J. (1974) Body fat assessed from total body density and its estimation from skinfold thickness: measurements on 481 men and women aged from 16 to 72 years. *Br. J. Nutr.* **32**:77–97.

Efthimiou, J., Mounsey, P.J., Benson, D.N. *et al.* (1993) Effect of carbohydrate rich versus fat rich loads on gas exchange and walking performance on patients with chronic obstructive lung disease. *Thorax* **47**:451–54.

Fitting, J.-W. (1992) Nutritional support in chronic lung disease. *Thorax* **47**:141–3.

Frisancho, A.R. (1981) New norms of upper limb fat and muscle area for assessment of nutritional status. *Am. J. Clin. Nutr.* **34**:2540–5.

Garrow, J.S., and Webster, J. (1985) Quetlet's index (W/H) as a measure of fatness. *Int. J. Obesity.* **9**:147–53.

Goldstein, S.A., Thomashow, B.W., Kvetan, V. *et al.* (1988) Nitrogen end energy relationships in malnourished patients with emphysema. *Am. Rev. Respir. Dis.* **138**:636–44.

Gurney, J.M., and Jellife, D.B. (1973) Arm anthropometry in nutritional assessment: nomogram for rapid calculation of muscle circumference and cross-sectional muscle and fat areas. *Am. J. Clin. Nutr.* **26**:912–15.

Harris, J.A., and Benedict, F.G. (1919) *A Biometric Study of Basal Metabolism in Man.* Washington: Carnegie Institute of Washington.

Heymsfield, S.B., McManus, C., Smith, J. *et al.* (1982) Anthropometric measurement of muscle mass: revised equations for calculating bone–free arm muscle area. *Am. J. Clin. Nutr.* **36**:680–90.

Hugli, O., Schutz, Y., and Fitting, J.-W. (1996) The daily energy expenditure in stable chronic obstructive pulmonary disease. *Am. J. Crit. Care Med.* **153**:294–300.

Lukaski, H.C. (1987) Methods for the assessment of human body composition: traditional and new. *Am. J. Clin. Nutr.* **46**:537–56.

Mancino, J., Donahoe, M., Rogers, R. (1993) Nutritional assessment and therapy. In: *Principles and Practice of Pulmonary Rehabilitation* (eds R. Casaburi and T. Petty). Philadelphia: WB Saunders, pp. 336–50.

Metropolitan Life Insurance Company. (1983) *Weight Standards for Men and Women.* New York: Metropolitan Life.

Muers, M.F., and Green, J.H. (1993) Weight loss in chronic obstructive pulmonary disease. *Eur. Respir. J.* **6**:729–34.

Scholfield, C. (1985) Predicting basal metabolic rate, new standards and review of previous work. *Hum. Nutr.: Clin. Nutr.* **39c** (suppl. 1):5–42.

Schols, A.M.W.J., Mostert, R., Cobben, N. *et al.* (1991a) Transcutaneous oxygen saturation and carbon dioxide tension during meals in patients with chronic obstructive pulmonary disease. *Chest* **100**:1287–92.

Schols, A.M.W.J., Wouters, E.F.M., Soeters, P.B., and Westerterp, K.R. (1991b) Body composition by bioelectrical-impedance analysis compared with deuterium dilution and skinfold anthropometry in patients with chronic obstructive pulmonary disease. *Am. J. Clin. Nutr.* **53**:421–4.

Semple, P.D., Watson, W.S., Beastall, G.H. *et al.* (1979) Diet, absorption, and hormone studies in relation to body weight in obstructive airways disease. *Thorax* **34**:783–8.

Wilson, D.O., Rogers, R.M., Wright, E.C., and Anthonisen, N.R. (1989) Body weight in chronic obstructive pulmonary disease. *Am. Rev. Respir. Dis.* **139**:1435–8.

6.
Physiotherapy

J. Bott

Physiotherapy
Department, Royal
Brompton Hospital,
London

Practical Pulmonary Rehabilitation.
Edited by Mike Morgan and Sally Singh.
Published in 1997 by Chapman & Hall, London.
ISBN 0 412 61810 9.

Definition, role and aims of physiotherapy

The Chartered Society of Physiotherapy, our professional body, defines physiotherapy as 'a health care profession which emphasizes the use of physical approaches in the prevention and treatment of disease and disability' (Chartered Society of Physiotherapy, 1991). It goes on to clarify physiotherapy skills and role with, amongst others, the following points:

- A physiotherapy analysis is based on an assessment of movement and function.
- A physiotherapy analysis takes account of current psychological, cultural and social factors.
- A central aim of intervention is to facilitate patients' maximum functional abilities.
- Physiotherapists teach and advise patients, relatives and/or carers on the optimal management of disabilities in order to enhance or preserve the quality of life for all concerned.
- Physiotherapists must be skilled in related educational and self-care approaches.

The physiotherapy role in pulmonary rehabilitation

It can be seen, therefore, that the role of physiotherapy and its central aim coincide largely with the aims and needs of a pulmonary rehabilitation programme.

For many years respiratory physiotherapists have been closely involved in the treatment of patients with chronic pulmonary conditions by helping patients learn to clear secretions, reduce their breathlessness on exertion and improve their exercise ability (Gaskell and Webber, 1977). It is interesting to note, however, that the same authors were advising their readers that 'older patients with chronic bronchitis or emphysema do not do well in classes and should be treated individually'. It would appear, therefore, that the greatest difference between pulmonary rehabilitation and previous forms of physiotherapy for respiratory disease is the group setting.

Although the physiotherapist, theoretically, is able to provide breathing retraining and exercise rehabilitation, this is not necessarily fully utilized or always available. The current trend for pulmonary rehabilitation opens this option for many patients for whom medication and medical support have otherwise been optimized.

The physiotherapist's role in the pulmonary rehabilitation programme will vary according to the local situation and the other team members involved, but is likely to include any or all of the following (Bott and Moran, 1996):

- Reduction of fear and anxiety.
- Reduction of breathlessness and the work of breathing.
- Improvement in the efficiency of ventilation.
- Mobilizing and aiding expectoration of secretions.
- Improvement in knowledge and understanding.
- Reducing (thoracic) pain.
- Maintaining or improving exercise tolerance and functional ability.

In assessment and exercise training

The physiotherapist is the health care professional most likely to plan and supervise the exercise training (systemic and/or respiratory muscle) within pulmonary rehabilitation. It is possible that he or she may also be involved in the initial assessment of patients' suitability for the programme and in assessments of quality of life and exercise tolerance. The individualization and assessment of the patient has been seen to be important within physiotherapy for many years: 'each individual patient must be carefully assessed and exercise within his limitations' (Gaskell, 1979).

As these topics are covered in detail elsewhere in this book, this chapter will concern itself with other techniques within respiratory physiotherapy.

Respiratory physiotherapy techniques

Reduction of breathlessness and the work of breathing

Inappropriate or excessive breathlessness (dyspnoea) is usually the single most important symptom to any patient with chronic respiratory disease. As the patient's condition progresses, this dyspnoea occurs with ever-reducing levels of exertion. The dyspnoea gradually becomes disproportionate to the level of exertion, drawn from the individual's past experience. This creates fear of the sensation, frequently leading to modification of lifestyle in order to avoid such exertion, and the beginnings of the vicious cycle of inactivity have insidiously appeared. Without some intervention, this spirals inexorably downwards until patients are trapped by their own unwillingness to perform any sort of activity that produces dyspnoea. This increasingly curtails both functional and social activities. It has been demonstrated that this reduction of activity in chronic obstructive pulmonary disease produces alterations in mental state, such as feelings of hopelessness, depression and pessimism (Burns and Howell, 1969).

Patients with hyperreactive airways have additional problems with unpleasant and frightening symptoms due to bronchoconstriction if venturing out in cold, damp or windy conditions, or sometimes in very hot weather. These symptoms may be more pronounced at nighttime and, coupled with fear for personal safety, this frequently limits outdoor excursions to daylight hours, and only then in good weather. Many such people become virtually house-bound and, if they live alone, this exacerbates a recluse-style living pattern. Living alone usually allows individuals to spend more time dwelling on their condition and unpleasant symptoms, and fear and anxiety mount, compounding the problem further.

Patients attending a pulmonary rehabilitation programme need increased self-efficacy in order to deal with these problems. Empowering patients with knowledge of their condition and a greater understanding of their symptoms is important. Likewise, learning simple techniques to control and reduce the work or breathing and the symptom of breathlessness is vital.

POSITIONING

The first step towards self-help is positioning; a simple, yet effective technique to reduce both the symptom of breathlessness and the work of breathing. Most patients with chronic airways obstruction adopt a pattern of shallow and rapid breathing, frequently with chest wall and abdominal asynchrony. Rochester (1991) describes the mechanism by which the patient with COPD produces this pattern to maximize ventilation, but at the cost of substantially increasing the work of breathing. Usually, skeletal muscle is able to contract most effectively from its resting length, although Green and Moxham (1983) postulate that in the case of the human diaphragm it may even be most effective at 125% of this. In patients with hyperinflated lungs, the inspiratory muscles are in a permanently shortened position and thus with a poor length–tension relationship. Despite some adaptation of the muscle to this shortening, such a diaphragm does not have the ability to produce the required large change in thoracic cage volume to effect inspiration; this alteration in volume, therefore, has to take place via an alternative means. This is with the shoulders elevated, utilizing contraction of the accessory muscles of respiration. Although by fixing the shoulder girdle in this way, thoracic cage volume is increased and ventilation is improved, the respiratory muscle oxygen consumption is increased and the overall net benefit is dubious.

Patients therefore need to be taught how to fix the shoulder girdle without increasing oxygen consumption, if possible, and to put the

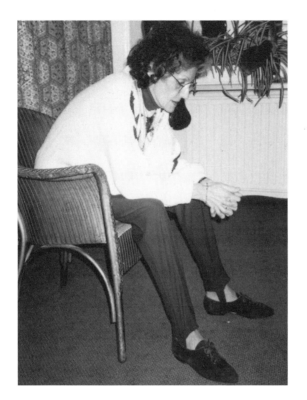

Fig. 6.1 The basic forward lean sitting position.

diaphragm in a more lengthened position. The forward lean sitting (FLS) position does just this. If a seat is available, sitting with the elbows or forearms supported is the easiest and most effective position. If no other form of support is available, the patient can rest the elbows on the knees (Fig. 6.1). Should a table or suitable height surface be available, resting the elbows on that may prove even more effective and comfortable (Fig. 6.2). For periods of extreme breathlessness at home or in hospital, judicious use of pillows can aid the effectiveness and comfort of this position. These FLS positions have been shown to be effective in reducing the sensation of breathlessness in patients with severe COPD and asthma (Barach, 1974; Sharp *et al.*, 1980), reducing the work of breathing (O'Neill and McCarthy, 1983) and the expiratory reserve volume and minute ventilation, without any worsening of the arterial blood gases (Barach, 1974) and reversing the paradoxical abdominal wall motion (Sharp *et al.*, 1980). Sharp and colleagues (1980) hypothesize that the benefits are most likely to be brought about by an improvement in the length–tension relationship of the diaphragm. The FLS position utilizes the incompressibility of the abdominal contents, forcing them up against the diaphragm, pushing it into a slightly more domed and lengthened position, thus improving its length–tension ratio and consequently its force of contraction. Moreover, the supported elbows fix the shoulder

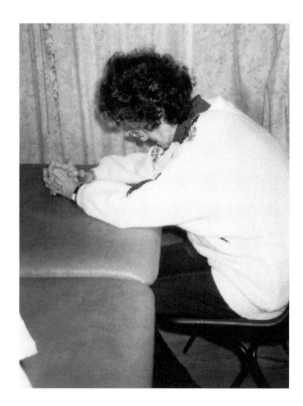

Fig. 6.2 Forward lean sitting position using a support.

girdle and optimize the thoracic cage movement. It may well be that, in addition to improving function of the diaphragm, the pressure exerted by the abdominal contents also passively reduces the hyperinflation of the chest to some extent. Not every patient will find the FLS position comfortable and supported upright sitting may be preferred by some.

At times during a patient's activities, there may be no seat available and the FLS position can be adapted to three standing versions with some success. If a wall or window sill, or other object at between waist and shoulder height, is available, the patient can lean and rest the elbows on this (Fig. 6.3). Alternatively, the patient may lean the back against a wall with the feet 45–60 cm away and allow the shoulder girdle to relax and the hands to hang free or rest gently on the thighs (Fig. 6.4). If preferred, patients may lean sideways against the wall with one shoulder firmly against the wall and with the shoulders again relaxed (Fig. 6.5). If a person's normal activity takes him or her to places where there are no such objects to lean against, a walking stick can prove helpful. The patient can then use the walking stick as a prop to lean on in a forward lean standing posture. If the patient gets considerably more benefit from the sitting position, there are walking sticks available with a small collapsi-ble seat at the top end (shooting stick) which forms a temporary stool. Some people may like using a shopping trolley with wheels, not only to

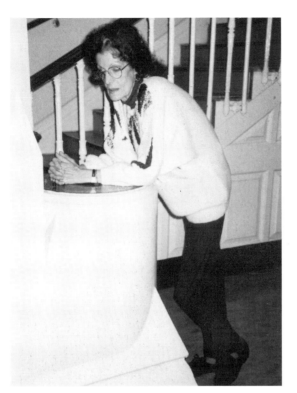

Fig. 6.3 Forward lean standing position using a support.

take the load of the shopping or other items to be carried, but also to provide the necessary object to lean on. Such trolleys make useful holders for a portable oxygen cylinder, if used.

Individuals may have adopted some of these positions naturally, but it is unlikely that all patients will be familiar with all positions. The physiotherapist needs to ensure that the patients in the programme try the positions and find out for themselves which ones they find easiest to adopt and which provide the greatest relief of their dyspnoea. This must be considered along with the patient's normal activity. The beneficial postures must be both effective and possible within the individual's environment. e.g. the forward lean standing position is not helpful if there is no suitable-height object available to lean on. The physiotherapist must find out about the patient's daily routine and environment and incorporate this knowledge into the teaching. Many patients are embarrassed or feel uncomfortable if demonstrating to others in public that they are breathless, and are most willing to adopt a posture that, in their eyes, will cause the least comment and be least noticeable to others. It is imperative for the physiotherapist to be sensitive to this. It is also helpful to facilitate a discussion between patients so that they may teach each other little tricks that they have learned and adapted. This passing on of knowl-

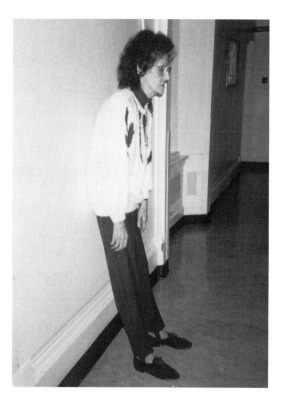

Fig. 6.4 Forward lean standing position supported against a wall.

edge and tips is one of the many useful features of a group rehabilitation programme.

It should not be forgotten that patients undergoing a pulmonary rehabilitation programme may suffer from an acute exacerbation of their condition from time to time. It is therefore important that the physiotherapist teaches patients positions to adopt when they may be more acutely ill. The FLS position over a table with cushions is one of the best for many patients but high side lying, again well supported with pillows, is frequently found to be comfortable (Fig. 6.6). For some patients with emphysema, the head-down position may bring additional relief (Barach and Beck, 1954) but is best first attempted in the hospital setting. In all such positions and when the patient is dyspnoeic, the position is most effective when the patient can relax and use breathing control at the same time.

BREATHING CONTROL

Over 30 years ago, Motley (1963) and Thoman *et al.* (1966) demonstrated that slow, controlled breathing to a predetermined speed produced an increase in tidal volume and a reduction in the arterial partial pressure of carbon dioxide ($Pa\text{CO}_2$). It was then recognized by physiotherapists that

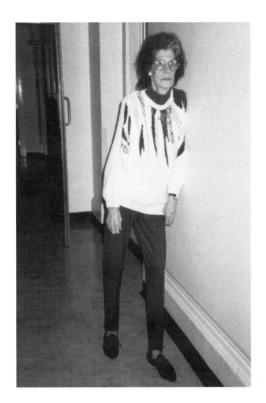

Fig. 6.5 Forward lean standing position supported sideways against a wall.

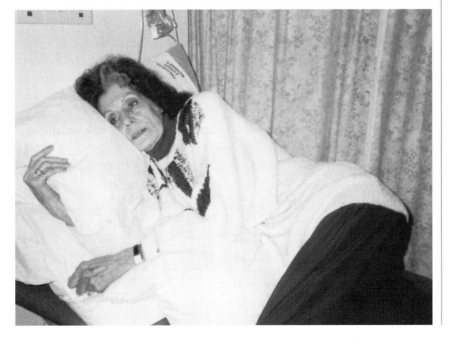

Fig. 6.6 High side lying position.

there were benefits to be gained from retraining patients' breathing pattern and that this would assist in the exercise training: 'after training in breathing control many of these patients will be able to tolerate graduated exercise reasonably well' (Gaskell and Webber, 1977). These views are still held today and one of the physiotherapist's most vital roles is to ensure that at a very early stage in the programme the patient learns control of his or her breathing and can use this control to assist with periods of extreme shortness of breath brought on by exercise or by anxiety. Along with positioning, breathing control needs to be taught as early as possible, preferably on the first visit. Breathing control at rest is defined as 'gentle breathing using the lower chest with relaxation of the upper chest and shoulders; it is performed at normal tidal volume, at a natural rate, and expiration should not be forced' (Webber and Pryor, 1993).

Previously, patients were instructed in diaphragmatic breathing, but with increased knowledge it has become evident that this is inappropriate. First, it is virtually impossible to isolate its action from those of the other muscles of respiration. Second, for patients with hyperinflated lungs and a diaphragm that is chronically shortened, contraction of this muscle will not produce the outward abdominal movement indicative of diaphragmatic excursion, and in severe cases may even bring about an indrawing of the lower ribs (Hoover's sign). It is imperative, therefore, that the physiotherapist does not persist in seeking large abdominal motion from such patients. Indeed, a recent study has demonstrated that taught diaphragmatic breathing increased the sensation of dyspnoea and the asynchrony of the chest wall, and reduced mechanical efficiency in patients with COPD, compared with their natural breathing (Gosselink *et al.*, 1995). Therefore, the emphasis should be on a comfortable, supported position, with the shoulder girdle particularly well supported, and the patient relaxed where possible.

Breathing control is easiest to learn when supported and comfortably seated, but is most useful when it can be adapted for use in any position and especially during activity. Patients should be strongly discouraged from rushing activities and the emphasis on breathing control during the activity ensures that the patient does not breath-hold, thereby optimizing ventilation. Timing the breathing to steps works very well when walking or climbing stairs, e.g. one step to breathe in and two steps to breathe out, or one for each, or any rhythm or pattern that suits that particular individual. Its use can be encouraged during exercise tests. However, in this instance it is important to ensure that if patients use breathing control on one test, they use it on all subsequent tests, or not at all, unless the test is to establish the effect of breathing control.

For all activities, particularly those requiring upper-limb exertion, such as wall press-ups or lifting weights of any kind, it is important to teach the patient to exhale during the exertion part of the movement and inhale during the relaxation phase of the movement.

The aim of breathing control is to allow the patient to function, albeit perhaps at a slower pace, but for a greater length of time and at a more comfortable rhythm, and needing less recovery time at the end of the activity. Teaching breathing control during activity may take the whole of a pulmonary rehabilitation programme as old habits die hard. Many of our patients may be so used to rushing activities to get them over with that this is one of the most difficult things for them to learn and to adopt. However, persistence with this technique is well worthwhile as even severely breathless patients with emphysema who are nearing the end of their natural life find breathing control a useful technique. Regrettably, little research has been done on this technique and its usefulness during activity.

PURSED-LIPS BREATHING

Pursed-lips breathing is a technique commonly adopted by some patients with chronic obstructive airways disease, typically those with some degree of emphysema. The lips are pursed during expiration, creating some end-expiratory pressure and thus maintaining small-airway patency. This technique has been shown to reduce respiratory rate, exertional dyspnoea and ventilatory requirement (Thoman *et al.*, 1966; Mueller *et al.*, 1970), and to increase tidal volume and oxygen saturation (Mueller *et al.*, 1970; Tiep *et al.*, 1986). However, pursed-lips breathing is postulated to have a detrimental effect on cardiac output by reducing pulmonary blood flow (Cameron and Bateman, 1983) and attempting to teach patients who do not spontaneously use the technique is not usually successful (Georgopoulos and Anthonisen, 1991). It is worthy of note that Thoman *et al.* (1966) observed that similar increases in tidal volume and reductions in Paco$_2$ were obtainable from slow, controlled breathing and hypothesized that these effects, seen in pursed-lips breathing, were due to slowing of the respiratory rate and not to the increase in positive airway pressure.

Clearance of secretions

Many patients attending a pulmonary rehabilitation programme will not have a major secretion problem for much of the year. However, it is not uncommon for patients to have increased sputum production during an exacerbation or infective period. It is important for the patient to remove these secretions as effectively and efficiently as possible. The role of the physiotherapist is to teach the patient to perform this activity independently, only using help from others if unavoidable.

In chronic airways disease there is usually some dysfunction in the mucociliary escalator, and sputum clearance is consequently impeded. Hypertrophy of the mucus-secreting cells and reduction in the sol epidermal layer lead to an increase in secretion production and viscosity. During an acute exacerbation, increased airway inflammation and bronchoconstriction with further airway narrowing compound the problem still further. Prolonged bouts of coughing are exhausting and many patients take steps to avoid it. It is not uncommon for patients with COPD to take cough linctus in the hope that this will stop them coughing. First, a good explanation of what mucus is, why we have it and its normal mechanism for removal must be given. The importance of its early removal and its role in infection must be emphasized. It needs to be explained that suppressing the natural cough is not a helpful thing to do when secretions are present and that the secretions need to be loosened and removed.

HUMIDIFICATION

In a review of the available literature, Conway (1992) argues that there is strong evidence for the addition of humidification, and that it can, in some instances, assist in the easier removal of secretions when added to a physiotherapy treatment regimen. It has been shown, in patients with reactive airways, that cold nebulized water can increase bronchoconstriction (Schoeffel *et al.*, 1981). Humidification is best delivered, therefore, in the form of either saline nebulizers, if the patient has a nebulizer, and/or steam inhalations.

Steam inhalations were once much in vogue and were considered clinically very useful. However, they became unpopular and have now gone out of fashion, due in part to the concern that patients might tip boiling water down themselves. A disposable system for steam inhalation has been developed with a flexible mouthpiece and lid (vapour inhaler, Anglia Vale Medical, Fig. 6.7), avoiding the need to tip the pot and ensuring maximum safety for the patient. At home, the patient can use such a device or a teapot with a cloth wrapped round the spout or a bowl. If using any of these, and in particular the teapot or the bowl, it is essential to remind patients of care and safety. They must ensure that the steam is not too hot for inhalation and that the receptacle is placed on a stable base and held firmly so that it will not slip (Fig. 6.7). Substances for inhalation that can be added to the water, e.g. friar's balsam, are readily available from the chemist. Their use is entirely personal preference. For the method with the bowl the patient places the face over the bowl of hot water and puts a towel over the head so that the steam is directed into the nose and month. It is more comfortable if the eyes are closed, particularly if substances such as menthol are added. Some patients find this method claustrophobic when they are dyspnoeic and prefer using a teapot or the commercially available inhaler.

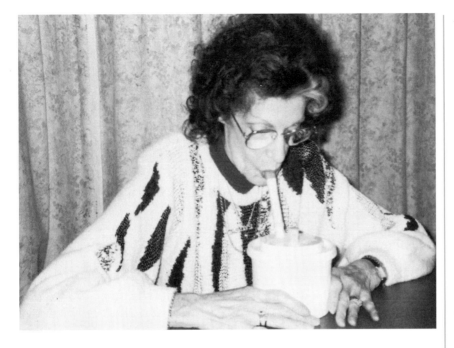

Fig. 6.7 Correct use of a steam inhaler (Anglia Vale Medical).

A hot shower can be effective and provides plenty of extra humidification, or, if the patient is able to use one, the steam emanating from a bath is equally helpful. In practice, however, many patients find baths difficult to negotiate and somewhat denervating. The increased pressure from a deep bath can exacerbate breathlessness for some individuals.

THE ACTIVE CYCLE OF BREATHING TECHNIQUES (ACBT)

This is a series of techniques or manoeuvres fully described by Webber and Pryor (1993), designed to assist with the independent removal of secretions with minimum effort. In patients with cystic fibrosis, it has been demonstrated to be an effective method of secretion removal (Pryor *et al.*, 1979), with no detrimental effect on oxygen saturation (Pryor *et al.*, 1990) or airway narrowing (Webber *et al.*, 1986). Its use is extrapolated to all patients who are able to cooperate in the clearance of their secretions. The term breathing exercises is less favoured today as exercise implies work and the aim is to clear secretions with minimal effort.

The ACBT consists of three basic manoeuvres. The core manoeuvre is breathing control, previously described. The second is deep breathing in the form of thoracic expansion and consists of three of four relaxed deep breaths. Last is the huff. The huff is a forced, but gentle, expiratory manoeuvre with an open mouth and glottis which utilizes abdominal contraction to expel the air (Webber and Pryor, 1993). A huff from full inspiration (high lung volume) will shift secretions from the proximal

167

airways only and should be used when the secretions can be heard to be loose in the airways. To retrieve secretions from the more distal airways, the huff should be performed from mid-inspiration (mid lung volume) and exhaled down to a low lung volume. The huff requires less effort than a cough and, when performed correctly, does not increase airflow obstruction. The action of the huff produces a dynamic collapse of the airways proximal to the point where the pleural and the airway pressure equalize. The lower the starting lung volume for this manoeuvre, the more distally the compression of the airway occurs, hence its ability to shift secretions from peripheral airways. The forced expiration of a huff should always be preceded and followed by breathing control in order to allow relaxation of the airways and prevent exhaustion. The combination of one or two huffs with breathing control is known as the forced expiration technique (FET). For a detailed description of the physiology of this technique the reader is referred to Pryor (1991).

The ACBT outlines all the techniques previously described, always interspersing huffs and thoracic expansion with breathing control. The cycle can be adjusted and accommodated to suit any individual and, depending on the patient's condition, emphasis will be placed on different parts of the cycle. For patients with reactive airways, longer and more frequent periods of breathing control may be required in order to allow relaxation of the airways and prevent bronchoconstriction. In other types of patients greater emphasis might need to be placed on the thoracic expansion to mobilize the secretions. If the patient requires extra help with the mobilization of secretions and needs chest clapping or shaking, these techniques would be added either by the patient or by an assistant during the periods of deep breathing.

The ACBT should be continued with the modifications as described above until either two huffs to a low lung volume are dry-sounding and non-productive (Pryor, 1991), or until the patient is too tired to continue. The sequence of techniques is designed to be used independently by the patient and can be performed in any position. For many patients, sitting may well be adequate when there are minimal secretions, but it can be performed easily in any postural drainage position should there be more secretions to remove.

AUTOGENIC DRAINAGE

Autogenic drainage is another method of independent secretion removal (David, 1991), designed originally in Belgium by Chevaillier, for use with asthmatic children. There seem to be two methods of performing the technique: the original method and an adaptation from Germany. The former consists of precise and carefully taught respirations at different lung volumes in a preset pattern performed by the patient. There are three specific phases: unstick (to loosen secretions), collect (to move the secretions centrally), and evacuate (expectoration). The three phases involve breathing at low, medium and high lung volumes respectively and cough is suppressed until the patient feels that the secretions are in the proximal airways. The German method is less rigid.

Autogenic drainage can take from 10 to 20 h of instruction, with additional sessions as required (David, 1991). Research has shown variable results with this technique, although a recent study has demonstrated this technique to be as effective and as acceptable as ACBT in patients with cystic fibrosis (Miller *et al.*, 1995).

POSTURAL DRAINAGE

Postural drainage (or gravity-assisted positioning) has been used for many years now for the clearance of secretions (Gaskell and Webber, 1977). These positions utilize the angle of the airways within the bronchial tree so that each and every segment of the lung can be drained if necessary. These positions were the mainstay of chest physiotherapy for many years, along with chest percussion (clapping), and have been found to be effective when the patient has secretions in excess of 20 g/day (Sutton *et al.*, 1983). These drainage positions are frequently an essential part of treatment for patients with bronchiectasis or localized chest conditions and in whom the secretions respond to the effect of gravity. When secretions are widespread throughout the lung fields and draining all segments would be impractical, the positions are modified to incorporate as many lung segments as possible and may end up just as alternate side lying, as flat as possible. Whether or not to incorporate head-down tipping will depend on the patient's response to this position. In cases of extremely viscous secretions or very small quantities, these techniques are now considered unnecessary (Webber and Pryor, 1993). However, each patient must be assessed and the appropriate treatment method instituted according to his or her needs.

CHEST CLAPPING

Chest clapping remains a controversial technique, both within medicine and within physiotherapy. Webber *et al.* (1985) evaluated self chest clapping with postural drainage and ACBT in stable patients with cystic fibrosis. There was no difference in the weight of sputum expectorated between the days patients performed self-clapping and the days when they performed postural drainage and ACBT alone. Gallon (1991) evaluated chest clapping with an assistant in 9 patients with hypersecretory lung disease due to bronchiectasis or hypogammaglobulinaemia. Treatments with and without chest clapping during postural drainage were randomized. Although there was no difference in the total weight of sputum expectorated, as with the Webber study, chest clapping increased the rate of sputum production, and most of the patients expressed a subjective preference for the treatments with the clapping included.

For a patient with a chronic hypersecretory lung disorder who has to perform chest physiotherapy daily, and possibly several times a day, the duration of the treatment is of paramount importance, to allow patients maximum time to get on with their own life. However, the necessity for an assistant removes some independence from the patient. For the moment, therefore, it seems reasonable, given the lack of conclusive evidence either way, that if a particular patient finds benefit from chest clapping it should be included in the treatment regime and if no benefit is found, it should be excluded. Whether the clapping is performed by the patient or a helper will depend on the patient's physical capabilities, the presence or absence of a helper and the patient's preference. Whether or not to incorporate chest clapping may also vary according to the patient's health status; many patients manage well on their own until an acute exacerbation, when they may find the addition of clapping helpful.

CHEST COMPRESSION WITH SHAKING AND/OR VIBRATION

The technique of compressing the chest on expiration with shaking and/or vibrations has also been used by physiotherapists for many years to assist in secretion removal (Gaskell and Webber, 1977). However, like chest clapping, they remain controversial techniques and have not been evaluated. These techniques are extremely difficult to study as it is not only hard to provide treatment with any one of these techniques in isolation, but every physiotherapist has a different method of performing the technique. The position of the hands, the force of the compression and the frequency and amplitude of the oscillations can all vary tremendously and objective measures of all these parameters are needed. There is room for much research here. For a patient in a stable condition the emphasis is on independence and, if patients find chest compression helpful, they can be taught to provide self-compression with or without shaking or vibration. When suffering an acute exacerbation, as with chest clapping, the techniques can be applied, if thought to be clinically effective by therapist and patient.

POSITIVE EXPIRATORY PRESSURE TECHNIQUES

Positive expiratory pressure, by mask or mouthpiece, provides variable expiratory resistance. It is titrated to give about 10 cm H_2O pressure for any individual, using a manometer within the system. It is postulated to enhance secretion clearance by maintaining airway patency and thereby reducing small-airway closure. It is used in the sitting position. For a fuller description of the technique, the physiological basis and a review of the relevant studies, the reader is referred to Falk and Andersen (1991).

The flutter valve is a small, hand-held device which produces oscillations and some positive pressure during expiration. It is claimed to loosen secretions for ease of expectoration and is gaining popularity in the USA and some parts of Europe. However, the flutter valve has been shown to be less effective in assisting with the clearance of secretions than ACBT in patients with cystic fibrosis (Pryor *et al.*, 1994*)*.

In the case of most of these chest clearance techniques, their evaluation has been done largely in the cystic fibrosis population. Extrapolating the findings to non-cystic fibrosis populations should be done with caution. However, until further research clarifies their efficacy, it is reasonable to use the simplest technique effective for any individual.

Education

Health education encompasses knowledge, attitudes and behaviour (Sim, 1993).

Increasing knowledge

Although formal education in the pulmonary rehabilitation setting is discussed elsewhere in this book, the physiotherapist involved in the care of patients with cardiorespiratory problems can fulfil the role of health educator in a wide variety of ways (Sim, 1993). Teaching independence, explaining the rationale for treatment regimens and giving advice go hand in hand with any physiotherapy treatment. Twenty years ago the physiotherapist *gave* the treatment to the patient. Today, this is no longer acceptable as patients need to be involved in their own treatment plans and decisions and, quite rightly, have far more autonomy than in previous years. The physiotherapist who wishes to help patients clear secretions, change breathing pattern, increase exercise tolerance or reduce fear and anxiety must inevitably educate the patient as well. This may take the form of education as to why they suffer from the problem, the various techniques and possible tools available to them, and all the related information required for them and their carers to feel equipped to perform these treatments and/or life adaptations.

Some of the other topics for education of the patient may also fall on the physiotherapist, should this be appropriate. Subjects they may feel equipped to discuss, in addition to breathing retraining and exercise, might be the pathophysiology of disease, lifestyle management, e.g. relaxation techniques, and when to seek medical help. Many patients with chronic respiratory conditions become reluctant to have frequent hospital admissions or feel they cannot bother the doctor. Some patients may choose, therefore, to tolerate a worsening condition and become seriously ill rather than seek medical help early. Patients can be alerted to various signs and symptoms that, if present, indicate that they should seek help. These include:

- Increasing dyspnoea.
- Change in sputum quantity or colour.
- Reduction in activity level.
- Excessive tiredness or sleepiness.
- Unaccustomed headaches.
- New or worsening pain.

It may be the role of the physiotherapist, in some settings, to assist in the teaching and handling of nebulizers, compressors, home oxygen systems and different medications and delivery methods. Should the hospital running the pulmonary rehabilitation not have an occupational therapist available to the programme, it may be the physiotherapist who educates the patient in energy conservation and tips for their day-to-day living.

Changing attitudes

Fear and anxiety play a large part in the vicious cycle of inactivity. Anxiety can be greatly increased if patients do not understand their condition or if their breathing feels out of control (Bott and Moran, 1996). They may have firmly held beliefs that they are not capable of certain actions or that it is dangerous to perform them. The reduction of a patient's fear and anxiety and the facilitation to change attitudes is an integral part of pulmonary rehabilitation. A vital part of pulmonary rehabilitation is to increase patients' knowledge and understanding of their condition and to increase their exercise ability and other skills (see above). These increase the patient's functional capabilities, which in turn increase confidence and social ability. All these factors are interwoven and, if the patient remains fearful and anxious, these functions will not occur.

Several other key factors are important to facilitate change in attitude and reduction of fear and anxiety. These are reassurance and praise, increased confidence and humour.

REASSURANCE AND PRAISE

One of the most important initial steps is to provide careful and sensitive explanation of dyspnoea and its causes and explain to patients that it is not harmful to them. We all experience breathlessness, but do not expect to get breathless just walking across the room to fetch our spectacles or a newspaper. This may be the situation for some patients and therefore reassurance of why this happens to them is a first vital step. Equally important and urgent to initiate are practical tips on how to alleviate this unpleasant and distressing symptom as soon as possible (see above).

The patient undergoing pulmonary rehabilitation will need constant reassurance: that tasks performed and consequent breathlessness are not detrimental to health; and that the grasp of techniques and performance are improving. Moreover, the general reassurance that a health care worker is in the vicinity reinforces this and patients with severe dyspnoea often feel better able to undertake activity initially within the rehabilitation setting. Between sessions and at the end of the programme it is extremely helpful for patients to know that there is someone whom they can contact when they feel anxious about certain things. Commonly, answers to simple queries and reassurance over the telephone may be sufficient. It may be a simple matter of reassuring them that they do need to seek medical help, or that whatever they are experiencing is normal. Listening to the patient's fears and concerns does much to alleviate them.

People find it reassuring to meet with others who are similarly afflicted and disabled. With sensitive facilitation patients can learn to talk to one another about their difficulties and distress and many find this of great benefit. With gentle encouragement patients will come to help each other and may offer practical assistance to one another, such as a car-driver giving a lift to someone without a car who lives nearby. Some patients find it helpful to have one another's telephone numbers and may prefer to phone another patient within the programme when they first wish to discuss a problem. Before this activity is embarked upon, however, it is imperative that the responsible health care worker ensures that any patient giving a telephone number is doing so willingly and not because of any form of peer pressure. The most useful programmes in the USA have some sort of maintenance programme and self-help support group following the cessation of the formalized hospital programme (Petty, 1993).

Praise for any help, improved understanding or genuine effort, as well as for improved performance, is a boost to self-esteem and cooperation.

INCREASING CONFIDENCE

One simple way of helping patients gain a little confidence within the programme is to allow them to share in the setting up of the equipment, making tea if that takes place or any activity that gives them a sense of purpose and helpfulness. Needless to say, a lot of praise is indicated when any of these activities are performed, although care must be taken to ensure that the patients who are unable to participate in this way are given praise for other reasons and not made to feel inferior in any way.

Care must be taken to encourage confidence in the patient's own abilities and their own judgement of their condition so that they do not lean too heavily on the health care workers within the programme. This is imperative in order to allow patients to wean themselves off the programme when it has come to an end. It is important that, from the outset of a programme it is made clear that it is for a finite period and is available only once, if that is the case (patients unable to complete for health or personal reasons should be excepted). Without due care and consideration for this, patients may have false expectations and become too reliant on the programme or specific health care workers. It is common practice in brief, interventional psychotherapy with a time limit that the issue of the sessions ending (termination) is addressed very early to minimize dependence and separation trauma (Poynton, 1991). Particularly for these reasons, some form of maintenance therapy or self-help support afterwards will help the patient handle this rather difficult experience.

FUN, LAUGHTER AND HUMOUR

Another useful way of addressing patients' anxieties is to make the programmes fun and to encourage laughter along with serious education and exercise so that patients can find humour in their difficulties. Again, this must be handled with enormous care and sensitivity. The group dynamics of every single pulmonary rehabilitation group will vary and the health care worker must remain attuned to this and safeguard the patients who do not readily join in or who prefer not to share in humour. Their own particular anxieties may be best relieved by quiet one-to-one conversation in the corner of the allocated room. It is imperative during all the sessions that patients with hearing or visual difficulties are catered for so that they do not miss out on vital information and sharing.

Modifying behaviour

Behaviour can be modified by learning. The increased skills a patient acquires in, for example, physical exercise or breathing control can increase knowledge and produce a gradual shift in attitude. Thus they are all interrelated. The separate physiotherapy activities are covered above and other topics are discussed elsewhere in this book.

Pain and stiffness reduction

Traditionally, physiotherapists are associated with the treatment of joint and muscle pain and stiffness. It is very likely, therefore, that the physiotherapist is the person to whom the patient will turn with such problems. It is important that the physiotherapist makes an assessment of the patient's problem and, if able, deals with it as appropriate. If it is a minor problem, this may be possible within the pulmonary rehabilitation setting. In particular, many patients with chronic respiratory conditions experience joint or thoracic cage pain or immobility. This should be addressed routinely, to some degree, and incorporated as an important component of any exercise programme.

The physiotherapist may prefer to see the patient on an individual basis for treatment of a specific problem. Most physiotherapists are probably familiar with treatments such as deep frictions, specific exercise, massage, posture correction, heat and transcutaneous electrical nerve stimulation. However, medicine and physiotherapy have advanced so far that it is likely that physiotherapists in full-time respiratory care may not be up to date with all the techniques available to them for dealing with the diagnosis and treatment of musculoskeletal pain. Should the physiotherapist not have the requisite skills to deal with the problem, or even make the diagnosis, he or she should not hesitate in referring the patient on to a colleague who does. Potentially of some importance to this patient group is the use of manual techniques (Vibekk, 1991) and acupuncture for thoracic pain and stiffness. This chapter will not attempt to cover any of the modern techniques used in the treatment of musculoskeletal conditions and for details of the physiotherapy diagnostic and treatment techniques, the reader is referred to appropriate textbooks and papers on those topics.

Even if the physiotherapist feels unable to deal with specific musculoskeletal problems, it is important that within the rehabilitation programme the physiotherapist is able to assess whether this problem inhibits the patient's participation in such a programme. If so, the problem must be dealt with as swiftly as possible. It may be appropriate that the patient's musculoskeletal condition is treated first and the patient joins the programme at a later date when more able to participate. It is very important that the physiotherapist looking after patients within a pulmonary rehabilitation programme knows what is limiting the patient's function, whether respiratory, cardiac or musculoskeletal. If the physiotherapist is concerned about pain that does not appear to be musculoskeletal in origin, such as chest pain or dizziness, he or she must refer the patient to a physician as soon as possible. It would be important in this instance that the patient is seen before exercise is next attempted.

Accessory equipment

It may be the physiotherapist's role to assist patients with equipment related to their disorder. Traditionally, it is the physiotherapist who selects and instructs patients in the use of the walking aid most appropriate to their disability. For the severely breathless patient, such aids may be used to increase mobility even in the absence of musculoskeletal disorders. Commonly used aids are walking sticks and frames (for discussion of the use of a walking stick for breathlessness, see the section on positioning, above). However, the patient with severe airways obstruction does not find the classic walking frame easy to use because of the need to lift it up with each step. More appropriate for this patient group are rollator frames, which can be pushed along. If the traditional-height frame is used, care must be taken to ensure that the patient does not grip the handles too firmly and reinforce arm and shoulder tension that the programme is trying to help them reduce. For this reason, the high rollator frame with forearm rests is particularly helpful for breathless patients, as it enables them to walk in a slightly forward lean position with the shoulder girdle supported. If the aid is for support for breathlessness alone, sensitivity to the emotions surrounding the issue and personal preference should be taken into account.

Conclusion

In summary, the physiotherapist has a large role to play in any pulmonary rehabilitation programme, ranging from the initial assessment and specific education components through to the regular exercise training. The extent and scope of that role will depend on local circumstances and on the availability and expertise, not only of physiotherapy, but also of other health care professionals.

Acknowledgements

I would like to offer grateful thanks to Jenny Causey, Sally Singh, Lynn Nichols and Elaine McKay for sharing their thoughts on the topic with me and allowing me to see their programmes.

References

Barach, A.L. (1974) Chronic lung disease: postural relief of dyspnea. *Arch. Phys. Med. Rehab.* **55**:494–504.

Barach, A.L., and Beck, G.J. (1954) The ventilatory effects of the head-down position in pulmonary emphysema. *Am. J. Med.* **16**:55–60.

Bott, J., and Moran, F. (1996) Physiotherapy and NIPPV. In: *Non-invasive Respiratory Support* (ed. A.K. Simonds). London: Chapman & Hall, pp. 133–42.

Burns, B.H., and Howell, J.B. (1969) Disproportional severe breathlessness in chronic bronchitis. *Q. J. Med.* **38**:277–94.

Cameron, I.R., and Bateman, N.T. (1983) *Respiratory Disorders*. London: Edward Arnold, p. 75.

Chartered Society of Physiotherapy. (1991) *Curriculum of Study*. London: CSP, pp. 12–13.

Conway, J.H. (1992) The effects of humidification for patients with chronic airways disease. *Physiotherapy* **78**:97–101.

David, A. (1991) Autogenic drainage – the German approach. In: *International Perspectives in Physical Therapy. 7: Respiratory Care* (ed. J.A. Pryor). Edinburgh: Churchill Livingstone, pp. 65–78.

Falk, M., and Andersen, J.B. (1991) Positive expiratory pressure (PEP) mask. In: *International Perspectives in Physical Therapy. 7: Respiratory Care* (ed. J.A. Pryor). Edinburgh: Churchill Livingstone, pp. 51–63.

Gallon, A. (1991) Evaluation of chest percussion in the treatment of patients with copious sputum production. *Respir. Med.* **85**:45–51.

Gaskell, D.V. (1979) Chronic bronchitis, emphysema and asthma. In: *Cash's Textbook of Chest, Heart and Vascular Disorders for Physiotherapists* (ed. P.A. Downier). London: Faber & Faber, pp. 231–48.

Gaskell, D.V., and Webber, B.A. (1977) *The Brompton Hospital Guide to Chest Physiotherapy*, 3rd edn. Oxford: Blackwell, pp. 78–83.

Georgopoulos, D., and Anthonisen, N.R. (1991) Symptoms and signs of COPD. In: *Chronic Obstructive Pulmonary Disease* (ed. N.S. Cherniack). Philadelphia, PA: WB Saunders, p. 357.

Gosselink, R.A.A.M., Wagenaar, R.C., Rijswijk, H., *et al.* (1995) Diaphragmatic breathing reduces efficiency of breathing in patients with chronic obstructive pulmonary disease. *Am. J. Respir. Crit. Care Med.* **151**:1136–42.

Green, M., and Moxham, J. (1983) Respiratory muscles. In: *Recent Advances in Respiratory Medicine* (eds D.C. Flenley and T.L. Petty). Edinburgh: Churchill Livingstone, pp. 1–20.

Miller, S., Hall, D.O., Clayton, C.B., and Nelson, R. (1995) Autogenic drainage and the active cycle of breathing techniques. *Thorax*; **50**:165–9.

Motley, H.L. (1963) The effects of slow, deep breathing on the blood gas exchange in emphysema. *Am. Rev. Respir. Dis.* **88**:485–92.

Mueller, R.E., Petty, T.L., and Filley, G.F. (1970) Ventilation and arterial blood gas changes induced by pursed lips breathing. *J. Appl. Physiol.* **28**:784–9.

O'Neill, S., and McCarthy, D.S. (1983) Postural relief of dyspnoea in severe chronic airflow limitation. *Thorax* **38**:595–600.

Petty, T.L. (1993) Pulmonary rehabilitation in chronic respiratory insufficiency: 1 – Pulmonary rehabilitation in perspective: historical roots, present status, and future projections. *Thorax* **48**:855–62.

Poynton, A.M. (1991) Basic treatment procedures. In: *Cognitive–Analytic Therapy: Active Participation in Change. A New Integration in Brief Psychotherapy* (ed. A. Ryle). Chichester: John Wiley, pp. 42–3.

Pryor, J.A. (1991) The forced expiration technique. In: *International Perspectives in Physical Therapy. 7: Respiratory Care* (ed. J.A. Pryor). Edinburgh: Churchill Livingstone, pp. 79–98.

Pryor, J.A., Webber, B.A., Hodson, M.E., and Batten, J.C. (1979) Evaluation of the forced expiration technique as an adjunct to postural drainage in the treatment of cystic fibrosis. *Br. Med. J.* **2**:417–18.

Pryor, J.A., Webber, B.A., and Hodson, M.E. (1990) Effect of chest physiotherapy on oxygen saturation in patients with cystic fibrosis. *Thorax* **45**:77.

Pryor, J.A., Webber, B.A., Hodson, M.E., and Warner, J.O. (1994) The Flutter VRP1 as an adjunct to chest physiotherapy in cystic fibrosis. *Respir. Med.* **88**:677–81.

Rochester, D.F. (1991) Effects of COPD on the respiratory muscles. In: *Chronic Obstructive Pulmonary Disease* (ed. N.S. Cherniack). Philadelphia, PA: WB Saunders, pp. 134–57.

Schoeffel, R.E., Anderson, S.D., and Altounyan, R.E.C. (1981) Bronchial hyperreactivity in response to inhalation of ultrasonically nebulised solutions of distilled water and saline. *Br. Med. J.* **283**:1285–7.

Sharp, J.T., Drutz, W.S., Moisan, T. *et al.* (1980) Postural relief of dyspnea in severe chronic obstructive pulmonary disease. *Am. Rev. Respir. Dis.* **122**:201–11.

Sim, J. (1993) Communication, counselling and health education. In: *Physiotherapy for Respiratory and Cardiac Problems* (eds B.A. Webber and J.A. Pryor). Edinburgh: Churchill Livingstone, pp. 173–86.

Sutton, P.P., Parker, R.A., Webber, B.A. *et al.* (1983) Assessment of the forced expiration technique, postural drainage and directed coughing in chest physiotherapy. *Eur. J. Respir. Dis.* **64**:62–8.

Thoman, R.L., Stoker, G.L., and Ross, J.C. (1966) The efficacy of pursed-lips breathing in patients with chronic obstructive pulmonary disease. *Am. Rev. Respir. Dis.* **93**:100–106.

Tiep, B.L., Burns, M., Kao, D. *et al.* (1986) Pursed lips breathing training using ear oximetry. *Chest* **90**:218–21.

Vibekk, P. (1991) Chest mobilisation and respiratory function. In: *International Perspectives in Physical Therapy. 7: Respiratory Care* (ed. J.A. Pryor). Edinburgh: Churchill Livingstone, pp. 103–19.

Webber, B.A. and Pryor, J.A. (1993) Physiotherapy skills: techniques and adjuncts. In: *Physiotherapy for Respiratory and Cardiac Problems* (eds B.A. Webber, and J.A. Pryor). Edinburgh: Churchill Livingstone, pp. 113–71.

Webber, B.A., Parker, R., Hofmeyr, J.L., and Hodson, M. (1985) Evaluation of self-percussion during postural drainage using the forced expiration technique. *Physiother. Pract.* **1**:42–5.

Webber, B.A., Hofmeyr, J.L., Morgan, M.D.L., and Hodson, M.E. (1986) Effects of postural drainage, incorporating the forced expiration technique, on pulmonary function in cystic fibrosis. *Br. J. Dis. Chest* **80**:353–9.

7. Lifestyle management: relaxation, coping, sex, benefits and travel

S. Gibson

Department of
Occupational Therapy,
Hinckley Sunny-Side
Hospital, Hinckley

Practical Pulmonary Rehabilitation.
Edited by Mike Morgan and Sally Singh.
Published in 1997 by Chapman & Hall, London.
ISBN 0 412 61810 9.

When faced with a chronic illness it becomes necessary to look carefully with the individuals concerned at their lifestyle in order to maximize their quality of life whilst minimizing the symptoms of the disease. This is no different in the case of chronic obstructive pulmonary disease (COPD).

The basic philosophy of occupational therapy is that:

- Activity is fundamental to well-being.
- People are individuals and inherently different from each other.
- Where occupational performance has been interrupted a person can, by being active, develop the adaptive skills required to restore, maintain or acquire function.

It seems wholly appropriate for this area of intervention to be carried out by an occupational therapist (OT).

Before starting treatment a model of practice needs to be adopted – 'an organizing technique designed to assist in categorizing ideas and structuring approaches to thinking about complex problems' (Hurff, 1985, cited in Kielhofner, 1985). This may be particularly useful to therapists new to the field or to the profession.

A good model is congruous with the occupational therapy philosophy, is applicable to the field of practice, describes each step in the process of intervention and states the methods and media that are appropriate for use. It provides a useful checklist, thereby ensuring that no applicable area is overlooked.

The model of human occupation described by Kielhofner in 1985 is one that is compatible with the philosophy of occupational therapy and is flexible enough to meet the needs of individuals with COPD. It also complements the work of other disciplines. Figure 7.1 outlines this model in more detail.

The focus of treatment is to enable individuals to manage their lifestyle in such a way as to achieve and maintain the optimal level of functioning throughout the disease process, i.e. to be able to engage in a balanced routine of work, play and daily living tasks within their environment and appropriate to their disabilities and their developmental level.

In order to engage clients in appropriate lifestyle management the therapist must have a clear understanding of the following:

- The nature of COPD.
- The implications for activity.
- Any risks involved and how to minimize or eliminate these.
- The nature of the medical interventions.
- The contributions of the other members of the multidisciplinary team.

From this information the therapist will then have an indication of the possible performance deficits of the individual.

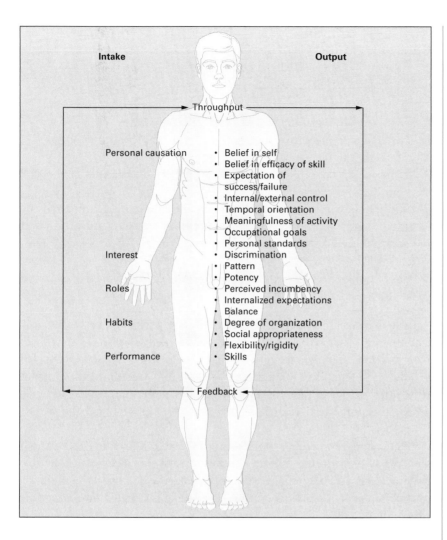

Intake

Output

Throughput

Personal causation
- Belief in self
- Belief in efficacy of skill
- Expectation of success/failure
- Internal/external control
- Temporal orientation
- Meaningfulness of activity
- Occupational goals
- Personal standards

Interest
- Discrimination
- Pattern
- Potency

Roles
- Perceived incumbency
- Internalized expectations
- Balance

Habits
- Degree of organization
- Social appropriateness
- Flexibility/rigidity

Performance
- Skills

Feedback

Fig. 7.1 The Kielhofner model of human occupation.

In addition, as clients will have patterns of behaviour they wish to attain or retain, and environments that they wish to enter or to which they want to return, the OT needs to be aware of patients' life roles and daily routines, as well as how they view themselves, their values and interests. This awareness, together with an understanding of their cultural background and the attitudes to disability, disease and health of those around them, can greatly affect the choice of intervention.

The knowledge gained from the above will indicate which needs require attention, thereby providing a focus for treatment and indicating the types of goals to be set. As COPD is a progressive lifelong illness, the individual is facing a life which needs to contain some achievement and quality whilst coping with the disease process and its effects on function.

The effect of COPD on performance

This is dealt with in more detail elsewhere in this book but, to summarize, the effects of COPD are as follows:

- Dyspnoea on exertion, in particular in severe cases.
- Muscular impairment resulting from reduced physical activity.
- Increased fatigue when carrying out an activity.
- Increased susceptibility to infection which exacerbates the COPD symptoms.
- Where hypoxaemia and sleep apnoea are experienced, impaired cognitive function with regard to attention, concentration, complex problem solving and the short-term recall of verbal and spatial information can result (Casaburi and Petty, 1993).
- Where pulmonary hypertension is present, angina-like chest pain may be experienced.

Disturbances as outlined above affect the performance of the individual in self-care, work and leisure. As the disease progresses, process skills become increasingly important – the individual needs to be able to solve problems, use adaptive equipment and plan for and anticipate difficulties. Once these become impossible to carry out independently the individual may have to rely on help or cease the activity altogether.

Adaptation to this situation is most effectively achieved if patients are able to communicate and interact positively with others in their environment. In chronic disease information processing, judgement and other process skills are all affected by the individual's emotional and personality traits.

Effects of COPD on habits and roles

Habits and roles are developed on performance skills and, as these are disrupted during the disease process, this, in turn, means that established habits and roles inevitably have to change.

A **habit** is a collection of behaviours which form the regular mode of practice used to accomplish a particular task. Once established, these tend to be more automatic and autonomous, not requiring conscious attention, therefore allowing more efficient performance of routine activities. If a habit has to be changed it requires conscious thought and concentration until the new routine of behaviours has been learnt and established.

Therefore a person with COPD who has to adapt to performance limitations is faced with new demands where habits are concerned.

In addition, individuals with COPD who require hospitalization or periods of inactivity as a result of acute infections face a change in routine and habitual tasks may be interfered with or suspended. As these are no longer practised regularly, the ability to carry out these tasks in a habitual way becomes impaired and will need to be reestablished or relearnt.

As habits and performance skills are affected by the COPD process, there is a knock-on effect on the **roles** performed. The impact in this area will depend on the demands of the roles undertaken by the individual, who may be unable to maintain or return to them. It may mean modification of the expectations of the role, finding different ways to enact the role or a completely new role and, as most individuals fulfil a number of roles in life, a combination of the above may occur. Such role changes can be extremely stressful; the patients may feel a loss of identity and may believe new roles to be less important than their previous roles, e.g. the sick or invalid role, or roles may be lost altogether and a loss of self-esteem can occur. When someone believes that above all else it is important to maintain the work/homemaker role, the stress and effort in so doing may mean that he or she withdraws from other roles, resulting in isolation, poor quality of life and a shrinking personal identity.

Effects of COPD on volition

The effects of COPD on the individual's ability to perform tasks and carry out daily routines are easily apparent, but the impact on an individual's self-esteem, self-worth, values and interests can be devastating and may not be so obvious. It is vital that these areas are examined as it is only when patients recognize and adjust to the impact of their disease that they are able to cope effectively with their situation. The effects of COPD on these areas are outlined below.

The COPD process involves increased breathlessness, fatigue and the reduced ability to perform skills. The resulting increased dependence on others and medication may result in the individual failing to develop the necessary adaptive skills, leading to a loss in internal control. This, in turn, may make patients reluctant to participate in activities which require effort and further confront them with their limitations, as they believe that whatever they do they will fail. This fear of failure can be paralysing.

As COPD is a progressive disease exacerbated by acute infections which runs an uncertain course, it is difficult for the individual to anticipate the future and what goals are likely to be achieved.

The course of the disease may mean they are no longer able to carry out a task to their satisfaction, requiring a lowering of their standards and compromise. Again, this can result in a lowering of self-esteem.

As a result of the disease, the person's valued goals may be partially or completely invalidated. Focusing on future goals gives a purpose to current activities and, where this process is disrupted, those with COPD may lack a sense of who or what they are becoming and be unable to find a purpose for struggling with the problems imposed by the disease. Also, if carrying out an activity means discomfort, limited performance and taking care, this may take the fun out of the activity which in the past held meaning for the person.

This is the same for interests. In addition, the need to spend more time carrying out self-care and work activities, interspersed with rest periods, will limit the time available for leisure activities.

The environment

It is also necessary to examine the physical, social and cultural environments within which the individual operates as these will have a major impact on that person's functioning.

The physical environment may present a number of difficulties to the person with COPD. The architectural design of a building, e.g. one with steps up to and inside, one with high and low cupboards in the kitchen, dictates the level of energy required to function within its domain. Such features can interfere with all aspects of daily living. The tools necessary for daily activities are usually geared to the able-bodied and therefore individuals may need to adjust to new or adapted equipment. Equipment may be rejected because it is unfamiliar or if it is perceived as accentuating the handicap.

If someone is to succeed in maintaining or adapting to a changing situation, others around that person must adapt their responsibilities and roles accordingly. Those most affected by the changed circumstances of the individual with COPD are their family and carers. It is likely that beyond this group their social circle will be small and will diminish further as the disease progresses. This can be caused either by physical barriers presenting difficulty, e.g. physical access to a building, or by social barriers, e.g. where the person regularly met friends in the local public house, the need to remain in a smoke-free environment may prohibit this.

In their changed circumstances the individual will need to face new social environments, e.g. hospitals, governmental/bureaucratic departments (for financial support or other public services).

In addition to the pressures outlined above, those with COPD may also be pressurized because of cultural prejudices. They may be seen as unable to contribute to society, for example, if they are unable to go out to work or to carry out daily living tasks at home. Cultures often dictate what happens, where and when, e.g. it is a woman's place to be at home with the children, normal working hours are considered to be office hours, and deviations from the expected can lead to isolation.

So it can be seen that patients with COPD experience considerable pressures in their interaction with the environment which, if not recognized and dissipated, can result in the individual and those around them becoming overstressed.

The treatment process

To initiate the treatment process, it is necessary to focus upon ways of enabling patients with COPD to achieve their maximum potential. This is done by implementing the OT process outlined in Figure 7.2.

Assessment

This is a method of gathering information. As individuals with COPD are likely to experience difficulties throughout the disease process, it is necessary to examine their lifestyle in detail and to look at the environments within which they operate.

How assessment information is collected will depend on a number of factors, e.g. time constraints, access to the individual and their family/carers, the availability of assessment media, etc. Although baseline data will be collected at the first point of contact with the individual, information will continue to be collected throughout the treatment process to determine the need for adjustment to treatment goals. Table 7.1 illustrates the main components of an initial assessment.

Standardized assessments

The use of standardized assessments is encouraged because these have usually been validated within the treatment setting for a particular client group, thereby establishing recognized norms. Measuring a client's ability to function is extremely useful as it ensures the results are reliable when set against the norms, and this can be helpful in identifying trends and recording outcomes of treatment.

The assessment needs to be relevant and applicable to the area to be assessed. It also needs to be easy to use for both therapist and client, sensitive enough to detect the differences expected or desired and to recognize the fluctuation of performance evident throughout the disease process.

Table 7.2 outlines assessments which may be useful.

Lifestyle management: relaxation, coping, sex, benefits and travel

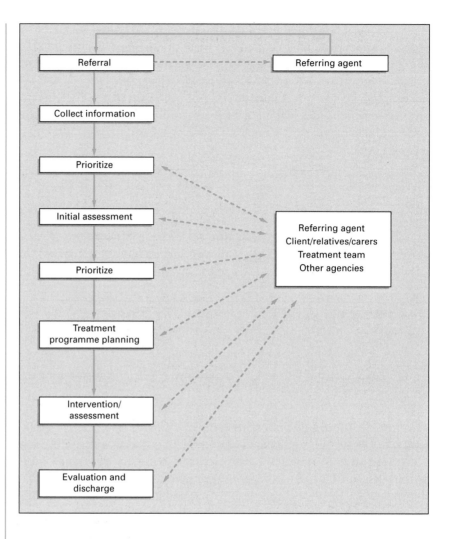

Fig. 7.2 The occupational therapy process. The process is flexible in that it allows, for example, intervention following initial assessment; regular moves between planning and intervention; and discharge at various stages in the process.

Defining the problems and identifying solutions

Tables 7.3 and 7.4 list the common problems identified by individuals with COPD and identify possible solutions.

Planning the treatment programme

Having identified the problems and suggested solutions, it is possible to group these together to form the main components of a treatment programme. These are:

1. Identifying and developing interests and goals which are compatible with values and the effects of the disease process.

Table 7.1 Main components of an initial assessment

Examination of the medical records	Provides information on the disease process, the drug regime, other disciplines involved and any medical precautions to consider in lifestyle management
Interviewing the individual	Provides the opportunity for two-way discussion and gathering information on the individual, lifestyle and living environment
	Provides the opportunity for the occupational therapist to explain his or her role in the treatment process
Interviewing the individual's immediate family/carers (either with the patient present or with his or her permission)	Provides further information about the individual and lifestyle, etc.
	Provides an understanding of the roles undertaken by the individual and family/carers
	Provides an understanding of the attitudes of the family/carers towards the individual and the disease
Standardized/non-standardized measurement of function	Provides baseline information on current functioning in day-to-day activities
Self-evaluation or self-rating tests	Provides an understanding of the individual's level of motivation, self-esteem and attitude towards chronic obstructive pulmonary disease
Home/work assessments	Provides information on levels of functioning and the individual's living/working environments

2. Maintenance of internal control through planning and problem solving.
3. Education in anxiety management.
4. Education in the principles of time management incorporating habits based on values and necessary treatment regimes.
5. Education in energy conservation.

6. Examination of current and future roles.
7. Maintenance of strength and coordination for the performance of self-care, work and leisure activities.
8. Provision of equipment to facilitate functioning.
9. Ensuring communication and interactive skills to enable the individual to negotiate for support and independence.
10. Identification of architectural adaptations required to home, work or leisure facilities to ensure maintenance of valued roles or interests.

Implementation of the treatment programme

The approach

In implementing the treatment programme, thought must be given to the approach to be taken. This must be compatible with the chosen model and in this instance a humanistic approach is favoured.

Table 7.2 Standardized assessments which may be useful		
Title of assessment	*Validated for*	*General comments*
Chronic Respiratory Disease Questionnaire (Guyatt *et al.*, 1987)	Patients with COPD	Self-assessment Administered by an interviewer Completion takes 15–25 min No problems reported on acceptability to patients
Canadian Occupational Performance Measure (Law *et al.*, 1994)	Rehabilitation patients including: Stroke Parkinson's disease Hip fracture and arthritis	Self-assessment Administered in the form of a semistructured interview Completion takes 20–30 min Although not validated with this client group, can be applied The patients have to be motivated and have good reasoning skills
Barthel Index (Mahoney and Barthel, 1965)	Neuromuscular and skeletal disorders	It is completed on observation of task being completed or from information from records It takes a few minutes to complete No problems reported on its administration It is widely known It is not able to measure subtle changes It has not been validated for individuals with COPD

Table 7.2 *Continued*

Title of assessment	Validated for	General comments
Functional Independence Measure (Granger et al.,1986, cited in Wade, 1995)	Rehabilitation patients	A global measure of function It is completed on observation of the task being completed It is a broader functional assessment than the Barthel Index and is more sensitive It has not been validated for individuals with COPD
Rand Functional Limitations Battery (Stewart et al., 1978, cited in Wade, 1995)	Measurement of physical health in terms of functioning in general populations	Self-assessment Administration takes approximately 10 min No problems reported in acceptability This is suitable for groups When severely disabled, other measures may be more suitable It has not been validated for groups with COPD
Older Americans Resources and Services Schedule (OARS) and Multidimensional Functional Assessment Questionnaire (Fillenbaum, 1978; Fillenbaum and Smyer, 1981, cited in Bowling, 1991)	Adults aged 55 and over	Self-assessment Administration takes 45–60 min Comprehensive assessment covering functional status in relation to social, economic, mental states, physical health, activities of daily living and current and past use of services Not validated specifically for individuals with COPD

COPD = Chronic obstructive pulmonary disease.

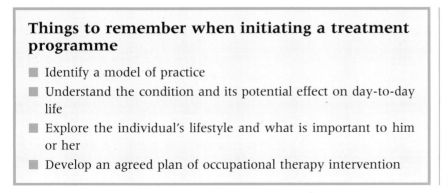

Things to remember when initiating a treatment programme

- Identify a model of practice
- Understand the condition and its potential effect on day-to-day life
- Explore the individual's lifestyle and what is important to him or her
- Develop an agreed plan of occupational therapy intervention

Box 7.1

Humanists take 'an holistic view of the individual and they prize personal experiences and openness to one's own feelings' (Hagedorn, 1992). Humanists focus on the positive and believe that everyone should be valued and if so they will respond accordingly. Humanists believe that everyone has the ability to control their own lives and that they will only change or progress if it is their desire to do so.

Using this approach with an individual requires the therapist to be authentic, honest and open and to display a non-judgemental regard and respect for the person.

Table 7.3 Defining the problems and possible solutions	
Problems identified include	*Suggested solutions*
Self-worth	
Loss of internal control	The provision of information on the disease
Loss of self-esteem	process
Lack of motivation	The successful engagement in meaningful
Increased anxiety levels	activities compatible with functional loss
	Appropriate training and practice in carrying out tasks
	The provision of adapted equipment to enable successful functioning, thereby facilitating control
	Training in problem-solving techniques
	Training in relaxation
	Always focusing on strengths and the giving of positive feedback
Values	
The inability to partake in past valued activities	Assistance in refocusing values and goals in line with current and potential abilities
Abandoning of valued goals	Goal setting, which stresses quality of life along with achievement
Values focused too much on achievement and too little on interpersonal relationships	Examination of standards of performance to identify and modify unnecessarily high or rigid standards
	Support and the opportunity to partake in valued activity
	Examination of values focusing on a shift to being and relating rather than doing values
	Involvement in measured goal setting

Table 7.3 *Continued*

Problems identified include	Suggested solutions
Interests	
The inability to pursue past interests	Provision of details as to where to find information regarding leisure activity
The reduction in pleasure when carrying out past interests due to the amount of planning and preparation needed	The exploration of new interests compatible with the level of functioning
	The adaptation of past interests to enable continued participation in these
Limited available interests	The involvement in daily time planning to ensure a balance between work and leisure
Lack of confidence in partaking in activity	The opportunity to practise skills required to undertake an activity to build up confidence in ability
	The opportunity to partake in assertiveness training

Other factors

How the treatment programme is to be implemented will depend on a number of factors such as time, the best location for the intervention, the best method of intervention, the availability of those requiring treatment, the involvement of others and resources available. Table 7.5 outlines these in more detail.

Methods of implementation

Below are outlined methods of implementing each component of the treatment programme.

Identifying interests and goals compatible with values and the disease process

This component of the treatment programme will run throughout the course of the disease and will need to be revisited at regular intervals, with subsequent updating. The achievement of this objective is fundamental to successful treatment, therefore it provides the focus.

To achieve the task in hand, it will be necessary for the therapist to develop a good working relationship with the individual and

Table 7.4 Defining the problems and possible solutions

Problems identified	Possible solutions
Roles	
The inability to function in past roles	The identification of skills and abilities for valued roles
Inconsistency in participating in existing roles	The identification of ways and means of partial role participation
Discrepancy between individual's and others' expectation of role performance	Suggestion of new or previously less important roles
	Patient and family/carer education to clarify the realities of the illness and help reduce patient/other expectation discrepancy
Habits	
Limitations in undertaking daily habits	Restructuring of daily habits to maximize performance and include other treatment regimes
Variability in function and performance ability makes stability in habits difficult	Education in time management
	Education in energy conservation
Skills	
Inconsistency in performance of motor skills	Teaching precautions to promote maintenance of motor skills
Reduction in ability to perform daily living skills	Ensuring use of specific breathing techniques
Disease-generated fatigue	Teaching new methods of performing daily activities and providing the opportunity to practise these
Angina-like pain on exertion	Education in energy conservation
The need to relate and communicate more as physical skills decline	The provision of adaptive equipment to facilitate the maintenance of activities guided by the patient's values and interests
	Teaching how to apply a problem-solving approach to personal situations
	Teaching how and when to ask for help from others
Environment	
Architectural barriers which hinder and prevent daily activities and disrupt routines	Evaluating and recommending modifications to the home, work and leisure environment
Attitudes of others around have a negative effect on the individual	Providing personal assisted devices
	Educating the family/carers on how to cope with problems experienced by the individual
	Assertiveness training

Table 7.5 Factors to be considered when implementing the treatment programme

Factor	Consideration
Time	Individuals' normal day-to-day routine
	How often they need to be seen
	How long they need to be seen for the task to be achieved
	When other disciplines are seeing individuals
	The best time for optimum performance, e.g. following drug regimes
	Does treatment need to be completed during an inpatient stay? Therefore treatment is time limited
	Is regular intervention throughout the disease process possible? This is the preferred arrangement
Location	Is it appropriate for the focus of treatment?
	Does it allow for privacy and dignity?
	Is it accessible where others are involved, e.g. family/carers?
	Does the location suit the patient's current medical condition?
	Will a simulated environment suffice? Are the skills to be practised/learnt, or transferable?
	Is it appropriate for the type of intervention?
Method	Will this facilitate the desired outcomes?
	Will this be an individual or group intervention?
	Is judgement impaired, resulting in a reduction in the ability to process information?
	When teaching new skills or adapting a skill, it must be practised for it to become habitual
	The need for all interventions to reinforce self-esteem
Involvement of others	Who does the treatment need to involve?
	The need to ensure that the individual remains in control of the future
Available resources	Not all areas may be able to be resourced and therefore priorities will need to be set to achieve maximum effect

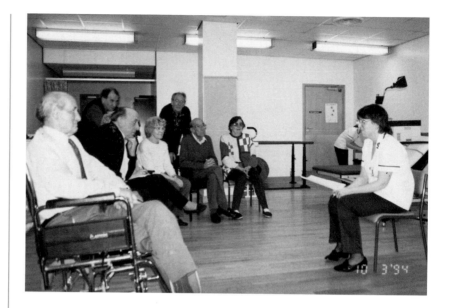

Fig. 7.3 Therapist and group.

family/carers, be skilled in eliciting and giving information and be aware of equal opportunities issues.

This component has to focus on the individual. But to reach the goal it may prove useful, in addition to one-to-one intervention, for the person to be involved in some group discussions/opportunities, e.g. self-help groups, group therapy, community and/or further education classes, and for relatives, carers, employers and/or friends to be involved as appropriate (Fig. 7.3).

Maintenance of internal control through planning and problem solving

The maintenance of internal control is again fundamental to the success of the programme.

The therapist is there to provide information to enable the patient to have informed choice, to advise and offer appropriate interventions, but ultimately the decision as to which course of action to take must lie with the individual.

As COPD is a progressive disease, the therapist should provide a method of problem solving for the individual to utilize through the course of the disease, for example:

■ Strategies for defining and analysing the problem.
■ A means of selecting priorities for action.
■ The ability to evaluate correctly possible solutions and select the most appropriate.

- The ability to plan and carry out the activity.
- The ability to evaluate the results, redefine the problem and plan new action if required.
- The knowledge of when and how to call in professional help if required.

Education in anxiety management

A number of studies have been carried out on the prevalence of anxiety disorders in individuals with COPD. The results have ranged from as much as 96% (Hodgkin *et al.*, 1993) to as few as 2% (Casaburi and Petty, 1993). Although the exact prevalence is unknown, it is clear that it is most common in individuals with COPD who experience dyspnoea. The anxiety is triggered by the dyspnoea, resulting in the breathlessness being exaggerated, leading to panic. Fear of this happening leads to a reduction in activity, so the individual becomes deconditioned and therefore more breathless on exertion, and a downward spiral ensues. Training in anxiety management helps prevent this.

Two approaches are favoured in anxiety management training: a behavioural approach and a cognitive approach. The former uses exposure therapy. Here, anxiety reduction occurs by exposing the individual to 'fear-eliciting stimuli and maintaining contact until the fear diminishes' (O'Sullivan, 1990, cited in Powell and Enright, 1990). In contrast, cognitive therapy is a 'structured form of psychotherapy designed to alleviate symptoms and to help individuals learn more effective ways of dealing with difficulties contributing to their suffering' (Blackburn and Davidson, 1990, cited in Blackburn, 1993).

Whichever approach is taken, the first stage in anxiety management training is to give the individual an understanding of the normal effects of stress and how breathing is particularly important for people with COPD, as in their case these effects are further exaggerated. This reinforces the need to keep anxiety under control.

Having achieved this, the person is taught ways of dealing with anxiety. In individuals with COPD it is usual to combine elements of both cognitive and behavioural approaches to encourage a balanced response.

Behavioural approach

A number of mechanisms may be used in order to help combat anxiety/panic. These are outlined below.

195

Relaxation

This copes with both muscular and mental tension and lowers the heart rate, reduces blood pressure, reduces sweat gland activity, alters brain-wave patterns and reduces somatomotor activity. This occurs because relaxation decreases the activity of the sympathetic nervous system and increases the activity of the parasympathetic nervous system.

Where relaxation training uses progressive muscular relaxation (PMR; Powell and Enright, 1990), i.e. muscle-tensing and relaxing exercises, the person is taught to become aware of muscular tension and how this can be released. Although the teaching of relaxation is a skilled technique, once learnt, patients will be able to recognize and deal with tension effectively themselves.

Therefore when using this technique with individuals with COPD, it not only helps in the control of anxiety but also puts them in control of their well-being. Often PMR is taught with the person lying supine on a mat, bed or carpeted floor; however, this can be taught as effectively or more so with the individual sat in an upright chair. This position is favoured for those with COPD as it enhances breathing and it can be more easily adopted as part of a normal day-to-day routine.

Distraction or diversion

A quick technique is given to use in any situation, e.g. thought stopping by shouting 'stop' and carrying out a physical action at the same time such as clapping; by creating mild pain such as digging the finger-nails into the palm; by focusing on a particular object in the room and studying it in detail; by reciting tables; by subtracting 7 from 100 and so on.

Different distraction techniques suit different people and it is essential that people choose a technique that works for them. It is important that this technique is employed immediately the symptoms of anxiety are experienced, before they get a hold on the individual. Again, mastering such a technique puts the person with COPD in control.

Graded exposure

This is particularly useful where the individual has used avoidance as a coping technique in the past. For example, the person with COPD may avoid leaving the house for fear of becoming severely breathless and being unable to control this situation. This technique involves facing situations which are the least anxiety provoking and progressing gradually to facing those which produce the greatest anxiety. It is called systematic desensitization and may be carried out with the involvement of a relative, but can be done with the individual alone. In the case cited above, the individual would initially leave the house, walk a short distance and return to the house. This distance would be gradually increased until the person is confident that he or she can remain in control.

Cognitive approach

This is based on the theory that maladaptive behaviour is a result of irrational and distorted thinking and that by altering this way of thinking, behaviour can be corrected. Examples of how this can be achieved are given below.

Self talk

This is where the person is taught to shift from a negative, self-defeating internal dialogue to one that is confidence building by substituting positive statements for negative statements when experiencing anxiety. For example, 'it's not going to be so bad'; 'anxiety cannot harm me'; 'I can cope'.

Stress inoculation training (SIT; Powell and Enright, 1990)

This is where people feel they do not have the ability to cope with demands made on them in a given situation. Here the person is given as much information and as many ways as possible of dealing with the situation and allowed to rehearse these using techniques such as role play before dealing with the situation in real life. This may be used in conjunction with the graded exposure technique.

Awareness of thought processes

Here the person is asked to remember a stress-provoking situation and to become aware of the thoughts that this elicits. The therapist then challenges irrational thinking, aiming towards more logical and positive thought.

Anxiety management cannot be achieved overnight: programmes often last months. The average session time is an hour, although this may be longer if it includes relaxation training.

Having assessed the person's level and cause of anxiety, it may seem more appropriate for this to be tackled in a group session rather than on an individual basis. This can be a more effective way of utilizing a therapist's time and it has been found to be the most effective way of achieving anxiety management (Powell and Enright, 1990).

Education in the principles of time management incorporating habits based on values and necessary treatment regimes

Time is a precious commodity which is finite. Being able to manage time results in considerable benefits to the individual with COPD, for example:

- Greater control over his or her life.
- The ability to achieve those tasks which are important.
- Reduction in stress.
- The ability to be proactive rather than reactive in facing long-term problems.
- A balance between personal, work-related and leisure activities, incorporating the necessary treatment regimes and rest periods essential to maintain optimum health.
- Increased quality of life.

So, having gained the commitment to time manage, the next step is to enable the individual to develop the right attitude of mind. Achieving this ensures that the individual will time manage with consistency. Fontana (1993) lists the following as essential to achieve the right attitude of mind:

- Clarity of thinking.
- Decisiveness of thinking.
- Single-mindedness.
- Good memory.
- Determination.
- A methodical approach.
- Punctuality.
- Calmness.
- Objectivity.
- Rationality.
- Leadership.

He states that we all have some of these qualities within us but we often fail to show them because they take effort. If, however, we make the effort, the benefits are soon evident. So if an individual is enabled to make a consistent and sustained effort to manage time more effectively, he or she will soon see the benefits, which will lead to more time-effective behaviour and so on.

It has been asserted that an individual's inherent characteristics play a part in whether he or she is a good time manager (Fontana, 1993). There is little doubt that this is true but an individual's life experience will also influence ability in this area. It is unlikely that someone will have been exposed to appropriate informal learning experiences or had the opportunity to learn time management techniques as part of formal education in order to develop and build on inherent qualities. Therefore until individuals learn and use the necessary skills, they will not be able to appreciate the benefits fully.

The steps to good time management

1. The first task in achieving efficient use of time is to examine how time is currently being used by keeping a daily timesheet. This should show how much time has been spent in personal tasks, work-related tasks, leisure pursuits and at rest.

It is also useful to state what the tasks were and whether they were undertaken alone or with others. In addition, indicate at the end of each day other factors such as the weather (which affects performance in clients with COPD), and the person's subjective view of the day – was it a good or bad day? Why?

2. Then collate the results under headings, to give a clear picture of how time is spent and give focus to the time management task. The following should be noted:

- How much time is spent in activity?
- Is there a balance between work and play?
- How much time is spent at rest? Is this interspersed throughout the bursts of activity?
- Is medication administered at the prescribed times?
- Are patients able to achieve all they feel is important to them?
- Have other interventions enabled time to be used better? For example, help with washing and dressing may enable the person to arrive at work on time.
- Are any areas of frustration/failure/concern identified by the individual?

3. From the information gathered, objectives can be set with individuals to enable, as desired, a better use of time, incorporating the tasks they feel are essential to their well-being and a balance between work, rest and play to ensure maximum quality of life.

4. Planning use of time is the first step in achieving the above. It is anticipated that spending approximately 20 min a week on planning can save up to 50% in time, therefore enabling the individual to have the space to be proactive and creative in preventing crises. Plans should continuously be evaluated to assess:

- Whether they were adequate, realistic or appropriate.
- Whether they were operated effectively by the individual.

- Whether others involved were cooperative and understood what was expected from them.

Fontana (1993) gives guidelines for planning which include the following, some of which have been adapted to suit the specific needs of individuals with COPD:

- Setting a time frame for each activity – identifying as accurately as possible how long it will take to achieve a task.
- Setting a deadline for longer tasks which may have to be done over a few days.
- Building into the plan rewards when tasks are completed. Obviously these will vary according to the individual.
- Making the plans as specific as possible by detailing not only when but how a task is to be achieved. This will ensure that when others need to be involved they have a clear understanding of when they are required and what they need to do, e.g. accompanying the individual to town by bus to purchase clothes.
- Setting aside blocks of time for a task and ensuring that these are interspersed with appropriate rest periods.
- Grouping similar tasks together, resulting in better use of time.
- Not attempting to do too much; concentrating on the things which have to be achieved.
- Delegating tasks which can be done as appropriately by other people, allowing patients to concentrate on things which need to be done by or with themselves.

5. As mentioned before, good time management relies not only on techniques but also on the individual being prepared to adapt to a new way of operating. Again, Fontana (1993) provides a good list of self-objectives. These include:

- Maintaining a positive approach.
- Being realistic when setting goals; setting for what you know you can achieve.
- Maintaining a healthy balance between work, rest and play.
- Knowing when to do what, e.g. doing less when it is extremely hot or cold and breathing is more difficult.
- Starting and finishing the day positively by planning pleasant tasks at the beginning and the end of the day, e.g. breakfast in bed in the morning and a relaxing bath before going to bed.
- Not putting off unpleasant tasks. Doing them sooner rather than later not only gets them done, but also prevents the nagging feeling when they are still waiting to be done. This often results in a real sense of achievement, boosting self-esteem.
- Not procrastinating over decisions.

■ Being proactive rather than reactive.

■ Aiming for excellence rather than perfection. Excellence is often achievable, whereas perfection is not.

■ Not confusing efficiency with effectiveness. It is important to make sure that what is being done is worth doing and that it is done in a well-organized and time-saving way.

■ Finally by making time management a friend, not an enemy.

6. Also essential to good time management is the appropriate use of others. Delegation has already been mentioned but it is important to know when, how and whom to ask for help.

Treatment methods

Incorporating time management into a treatment programme can be done by working with the individual alone, or within a group or a combination of the two. The group method is favoured: the basic principles are given to a group, the individuals are encouraged to put these into practice and then return to discuss the results as a group. This enables a cross-fertilization of ideas and encouragement to the sceptics who perhaps doubt the benefits of adopting such techniques and therefore lack motivation.

Where time is at a premium, i.e. imminent discharge from hospital, it may only be possible to provide written material for the person to take home and apply. This is the least favoured method of treatment.

Education in energy conservation. Adapt it, don't subtract it!

Individuals with COPD often become breathless when carrying out tasks or taking part in activities, particularly as the disease increases in severity. This can often lead to their avoiding activity, resulting in a reduction in independence and ability and consequently a loss of self-esteem. An understanding of how to conserve energy can result in better forward planning and therefore enable the person to retain self-control and optimum quality of life.

Energy conservation can be achieved by adopting new methods of working, by providing equipment to assist in carrying out the task, by adapting the environment or a combination of all three.

Methods of working

Adopting time management techniques can also result in energy conservation as dyspnoea can be reduced or prevented by carefully planning and executing activities.

201

Where activities place an increased demand on the cardiovascular system, they should be spaced throughout the day, week, month and year to allow for maximum rest and recuperation in order for the system to function as effectively as possible.

Where necessary, tasks should be planned around the availability of others who can assist, and be carried out at the time of day when the person feels best. For people with COPD this is usually in the afternoon or following medication.

In carrying out a task the method used should be examined and adapted accordingly. The following can act as a good guide:

- Sitting as much as possible when undertaking a task.
- Breathing out when carrying out the most strenuous part of an activity, e.g. when vacuuming, breathing out when pulling the vacuum towards the body.
- Taking frequent rests during and between tasks, allowing the body to recover.
- Where angina is present, taking glyceryl trinitrate or isosorbide as a prophylactic before carrying out a strenuous activity.
- Interspersing heavy activities with light activities.
- Learning pacing – breaking down activities into achievable chunks.
- Taking into account external factors, such as the weather, before planning to carry out a task.
- Avoiding lifting, but when having to lift, holding the article as close to the body as possible and lifting by bending at the knees, keeping the back straight. This is good for the back and also prevents constriction of the chest cavity, thereby enabling the optimum oxygen intake.
- Pushing an object rather than pulling it, as pulling uses more energy.

The provision of equipment

The amount and type of equipment will depend on the stage of the disease and can range from a simple tap turner to a recliner chair, a stair-lift, an electric wheelchair to a scooter or hoist (Fig. 7.4). From experience, the most valuable pieces of equipment to maintain independence are:

- Bath board and seat.
- Shower stool.
- Towelling bath robe.
- Helping hand.
- Sock gutter.
- Raised toilet seat.

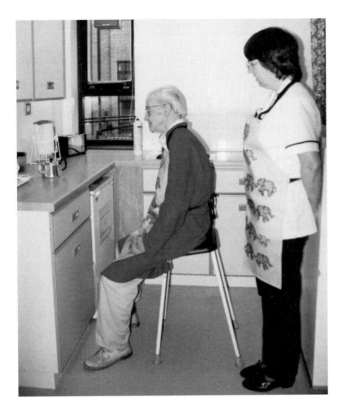

Fig. 7.4 Provision of
equipment: a perching stool.

■ Chair and bed raisers.
■ Perching stool.
■ Trolley.
■ Automatic washing machine.
■ Tumble dryer.
■ Microwave.
■ Freezer.
■ Stairlift.
■ Scooter for outdoor use.

Where intervention takes place at the early stage of treatment, careful planning allows the staggered introduction of equipment at the appropriate time and the provision of more expensive equipment which may not otherwise be an option, e.g., a stairlift or a scooter for outdoor use.

Adaptation of the environment

Again, how the environment is adapted for energy conservation depends on the stage of the disease. The most common adaptations are the introduction of grabrails, e.g. over the bath or on the stairs, and the reutilization of cupboard space to facilitate mid-range movement and eliminate stretching and bending. It has been known for individuals to be rehoused where additional complications are present, e.g. inappropriate heating.

Where major adaptations are a requirement, close liaison is necessary with the Social Services department and, where in place, joint working procedures should be followed.

Examination of current and future roles

Roles provide the structure to life and relate to status, social convention, culture and family life (Johnson, 1992, cited in Kielhofner, 1985). People with COPD experience physical limitations which frequently interfere with their normal adult roles. Changing roles can be extremely stressful for both the individual and those around him or her, as there are often different levels of expectation.

An adult may be required to fulfil a number of roles:

- Worker/breadwinner.
- Partner/spouse.
- Homemaker.
- Parent.
- Child (where involved with elderly parents).
- Friend.

It is necessary to examine each individual's roles, involving others as necessary to identify with the individual where changes need to be made and to look at how these are best achieved.

It is important that patients participate fully in this aspect of treatment to retain control over their future and adapt appropriately to increased limitations. Failure to do this inevitably leads to a lowering of self-esteem and decreased role performance, resulting in a greater dependence on others and a reduction in quality of life.

It is necessary not only to make the necessary adaptations to roles but also to ensure that role balance is maintained and, as COPD is progressive, it will be necessary for the person to adapt further as the disease progresses.

Sexual activity

This is a necessary part of living, as individuals are sexual beings even if they have not participated in physical sex for years. It is important when examining roles to address the area of sexual activity and yet, often because it is a sensitive subject, it is neglected unless raised by the patient.

It is particularly important that individuals with a chronic progressive disease such as COPD can feel able to explore both their own and their partner's needs and be given the necessary help. This is because their failure to perform in a normal way in their sexual role may result in them feeling unwanted, unloved and an encumbrance. Sexual intimacy can be a powerful antidote to the depression and isolation that can result from these feelings (Hodgkin *et al.,* 1993).

At the age COPD becomes apparent, people often feel unable to raise issues concerning sexual activity. This may be because they feel that sexual intercourse is for the young and that to be seen as still partaking would be socially unacceptable. However, for many, sexual intimacy remains very important, therefore it is crucial that individuals are enabled to share their concerns.

This sharing can be achieved by asking open-ended questions about sexual intimacy when exploring roles.

Any responses must be non-judgemental and it is important to ensure the discussion leaves the individual in no doubt that having sexual needs and feelings is normal. It is also important to pick up on any concerns conveyed and to use language that the individual understands.

For those with COPD there are three main areas of difficulty which need to be tackled:

1. Overcoming limited physical functioning.
2. A poor psychological state.
3. The effects of the medication.

Overcoming limited physical functioning

As with other activity, individuals partaking in sexual activity may be afraid that they will become breathless and not recover. If the person does partake and becomes breathless and has to cease in mid-performance, this is likely to leave him or her feeling unsatisfied and a failure, and may mean that he or she will stop any sexual activity. In overcoming these difficulties it is important to reassure patients that having sexual intercourse is no more stressful than climbing a flight of stairs and to give advice and guidance, such as to partake when they feel rested and to use positions which reduce exertion and pressure on the chest, yet produce sexual fulfilment.

It may also help to administer a bronchodilator immediately before intercourse or to use oxygen during intercourse.

A poor psychological state

People with COPD often suffer from a lack of identity and low self-esteem. It is known that these symptoms result in a decreased libido and ability to perform sexually. It is important, therefore, if the individual is to achieve sexual satisfaction for him or her to attain or retain self-worth. This can be done by enabling role fulfilment, as outlined earlier.

The effects of the medication

Medication used to control the symptoms experienced in COPD may also affect the individual's ability to perform sexually. If this is the case, this must be brought to the attention of the medical staff and a thorough review of the medication must take place and doses reduced or alternatives sought to improve the situation.

It is advisable that the partner is involved in discussions regarding sexual performance as his or her cooperation is likely to be necessary if sexual fulfilment is to be achieved.

Maintenance of strength and coordination for the performance of self-care, work and leisure activities

In order to ensure optimum physical strength and coordination, it is imperative that the individual undertakes regular exercise. An appropriate regime to suit the individual should be developed under the guidance of the physiotherapist involved with the treatment programme, and this is discussed in more detail elsewhere in this book. However, once established it is imperative that this is incorporated into the patient's daily routine as the successful implementation of such activities has a knock-on effect on everything else the person undertakes, enabling him or her to maintain optimum independence, optimum physical fitness and also a healthy psychological state.

Provision of equipment to facilitate functioning

Although the provision of equipment has been touched upon when focusing on energy conservation, it must be noted that this may not be the only reason why equipment is recommended or provided.

Other reasons may include:

■ To maintain optimum independence.
■ To ensure optimum comfort.

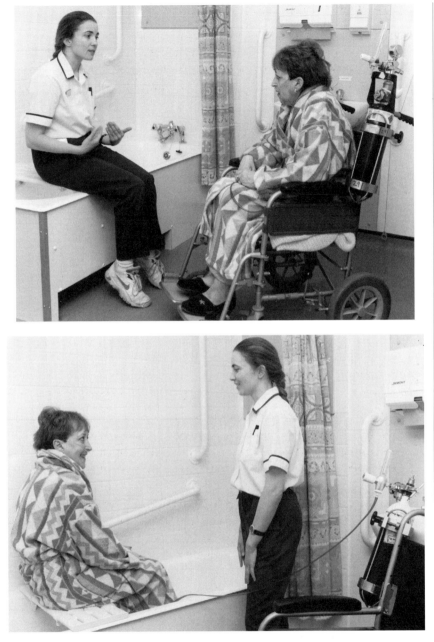

Fig. 7.5 Provision of
equipment to facilitate
functioning.

Fig. 7.6 Provision of
equipment to facilitate
functioning.

- To enable carers to manage the person at home.
- To ensure optimum quality of life.

It is important to be aware of the sources of supply of equipment in
the area as these can vary. Possible sources are:

- The hospital.
- The medical aids department.

■ Local charities.
■ Local retail outlets.
■ Direct from the manufacturers.

How individuals acquire equipment will vary. They may:

■ Be able to have the equipment on loan for as long as it is needed (from a charity or medical aids department).
■ Have to purchase the equipment themselves.
■ Have to pay rental.
■ Be able to get a local grant for its purchase.

It is important that the therapist is familiar with the local arrangements and to stress to patients the importance of being properly assessed before being supplied or purchasing equipment to ensure that it adequately meets their needs.

In some localities it is possible for the person to have access to a disability services centre or disabled living centre which houses a wide range of equipment for independence. It is imperative that all equipment is carefully selected. In particular, when choosing a large, costly item available in different styles, the opportunity to try such equipment must be provided without sales pressure. Where access to these facilities is possible, professionals are usually on hand to advise, although this may require the individual to make a specific appointment.

Ensuring communication and interactive skills to enable the individual to negotiate for support and independence

Communication takes different forms – it can be verbal, written or expressed using actions. All forms of communication follow a process: a message or idea is formulated; it is presented; and it is received and understood by the person intended. Ability to communicate is affected by a number of factors, for example:

■ Development.
■ Education.
■ Social contact.
■ Knowledge of the language.
■ Physical or psychological impairment.

In ensuring individuals with COPD have the necessary communication skills, other factors have to be considered in addition – those which may result from the disease process. These include:

■ Low self-esteem.
■ Reduced social contact.
■ Speech impairment due to breathing difficulties.

Low self-esteem

If throughout the treatment process attention is paid to ensuring individuals retain control over their future by being fully involved in the decision making and being given the necessary knowledge and/or skills facilitating the maintenance of self-esteem, they will have the confidence and the ability to communicate their needs clearly.

SOCIAL SECURITY BENEFITS

The importance of the patient understanding the disease process and approaches to treatment has been outlined earlier but an area which has not been covered is that of benefits. It is often because people are not aware of their entitlements that they fail to receive the available financial assistance, which may in turn limit the support they receive and therefore their independence.

A number of sources can be tapped to obtain such information. These include:

■ The hospital social worker.
■ Social Services departments.
■ Benefits agencies.
■ Local charities' organizational and self-help groups.
■ The Citizens Advice Bureau.
■ Local council offices.

Benefits are not only financial. They can include how to access equipment and local services, e.g. Home Care, Meals on Wheels, transport, etc.

As each individual's circumstances will be different because information of this nature is continually changing and the factors influencing available benefits are variable, it is advisable to seek out those who hold the fullest and most up-to-date information. Contact early on in the disease process will ensure that individuals can make use of all the opportunities available to them and enable them to negotiate with confidence.

Limited social contact

If this is addressed early in the disease process it is likely that an individual's social contacts can be maintained.

Encouraging the person to make contact with agencies and groups such as self-help groups results in the prevention of social isolation and provides a route to information. Local groups not only organize regular meetings of members; they often make regular contact by telephone, through newsletters and by home visiting as well as organizing social and/or fund-raising events.

Information on groups operating locally can be obtained via the hospital social worker or by contacting the main library or Citizens

Ensuring communication and interactive skills to enable the individual to negotiate for support and independence

Advice Bureau. Groups specific to individuals with COPD can be identified through the British Lung Foundation or Breathe Easy and if there is not a local group, considerable benefit can be gained by starting one.

Speech impairment through physical impairment

As the disease process progresses, individuals may experience communication difficulties as a result of a reduction in oxygen supply to the body. In such cases it is necessary to look at alternative ways of communicating. If this is addressed at an early enough stage, the necessary level of communication can be retained.

A way of addressing this is by using other methods of communication such as written messages, sign language or the use of technological equipment. Relatives and/or carers need to be involved in this process. A referral to the local speech and language therapy service may also be of assistance.

It may also be necessary to look at methods of raising the alarm should the person get into difficulty when alone. Personal alarm systems such as the Piper Alarm and Aid Call can be invaluable in providing reassurance to the person or relatives/carers that help can be quickly summoned. Both these systems are linked by telephone. There are others, such as pull-cord systems, which link to a local office. These are usually in city or sheltered accommodation and they rely on the person being mobile enough to reach the cord.

Identification of architectural adaptations required to home, work or leisure facilities for maintenance of valued roles or interests

This is the statutory responsibility of the local authority OTs who, under the Chronically Sick and Disabled Persons Act (1970), are required to carry out an assessment of the needs of individuals referred to them in relation to major adaptations of their living environments. They, too, advise the local authority housing and building departments where local facilities are being developed or adapted to suit the needs of disabled people.

Where it is known or expected that the individual with COPD will require alterations to the living environment or rehousing, it is advisable to contact the appropriate Social Services office as soon as possible. This will allow the planning and, where appropriate, grant applications to be submitted, avoiding delay and thereby ensuring that the process is completed as quickly and efficiently as possible.

Key points when implementing a treatment programme

■ Select an approach which suits
■ Take into consideration all the relevant factors which are likely to affect the implementation of treatment programmes
■ At the start prioritize goals to be achieved
■ Review these at regular agreed intervals and adapt accordingly
■ Record the outcomes

Box 7.2

Evaluating the outcomes

As has been stated, the desired outcomes of intervention are agreed with the individual at the onset of treatment as well as how they are to be measured.

The aim of evaluating the outcomes is to measure the effectiveness and success of the treatment. This is done at various stages during treatment to enable the following:

■ Assessment of the individual's progress in relation to the goals agreed at the onset of treatment.
■ A decision as to whether these goals are still appropriate or whether they need to be adapted in the light of new information.
■ A decision as to whether the goals can be achieved using the planned method or whether an alternative method should be used.
■ Referral to another agency to be made as appropriate, e.g. local authority OTs.
■ A discharge date to be set for the episode of care.

At the end of each episode of care it is useful to evaluate the total treatment, as this can provide a valuable source of information when and if the individual is re-referred at a later date.

Conclusion

It can be seen that by selecting an appropriate model, adopting a relevant approach, identifying with individuals their needs, planning and carrying out relevant and timely interventions, and evaluating the outcomes, it is possible to equip an individual with COPD with the necessary knowledge and/or skills to enable them to stay in control of their lifestyle, ensuring optimum independence and quality of life.

References

Blackburn, I.M. (1993) *Cognitive Therapy for Depression and Anxiety.* Oxford: Blackwell Scientific.

Bowling, A. (1991) *Measuring Health.* Buckingham: Open University Press.

Casaburi, R., Petty, T. (1993) *Principles and Practice of Pulmonary Rehabilitation.* Philadelphia, PA: WB Saunders.

Fontana, D. (1993) *Managing Time.* London: British Psychological Society.

Fontana, D. (1994) *Managing Stress – Problems in Practice.* British Psychological Society. London: Routledge.

Guyatt, G.H., Berman, L.H., Townsend, M. *et al.* (1987) A measure of quality of life for clinical trials in chronic lung disease. *Thorax* **42**:773–8.

Hagedorn, R. (1992) *Occupational Therapy – Foundations for Practice.* Edinburgh: Churchill Livingstone.

Hodgkin, J., Conners, G., Bell, W. (1993) *Pulmonary Rehabilitation – Guidelines to Success.* Philadelphia, PA: Lippincott.

Kielhofner, G. (1985) *The Model of Human Occupation.* Baltimore: Williams & Wilkins.

Law, M., Baptiste S., Carswell, A. *et al.* (1994) *Canadian Occupational Performance Measure.* Toronto: CAOT Publications ACE.

Mahoney, F.I., and Barthel, D.W. (1965) Functional evaluation: the Barthel index. *M. State Med. J.* **14**:61–5.

Powell, T., Enright, S. (1990) *Anxiety and Stress Management.* London: Routledge.

Turner, A., Foster, M., Johnson, S. (1992) *Occupational Therapy and Physical Dysfunction.* Edinburgh: Churchill Livingstone.

Wade, D. (1995) *Measurement in Neurological Rehabilitation.* Oxford: Oxford Medical Publications.

8. Disease education and medical support

M.D.L. Morgan

Department of Respiratory Medicine and Thoracic Surgery, Glenfield Hospital, Leicester

Practical Pulmonary Rehabilitation.
Edited by Mike Morgan and Sally Singh.
Published in 1997 by Chapman & Hall, London.
ISBN 0 412 61810 9.

The role of the physician

The majority of multidisciplinary pulmonary rehabilitation programmes will have some contribution from medical staff. This may vary according to the enthusiasm of the physician and the responsibility that he or she has within the programme. Usually the doctor will provide the classes on disease education and contribute to the advice given to patients regarding the technical aspects of their medical treatment. Even those physicians who do not formally contribute to a programme will unwittingly give some rehabilitation advice in their practice.

Disease education alone has not been shown to be sufficient to improve the outcome of chronic lung disease (Toshima *et al.*, 1990). However, it is likely that disease education stimulates interest in the programme as well as providing a knowledge base to ensure compliance

Models of medical participation in pulmonary rehabilitation

Direction of the programme

Lectures to groups

Joint assessment clinics

Referral of patients

Box 8.1

Table 8.1 Content and setting of disease education in rehabilitation	
Educational opportunities in rehabilitation	*Content*
Lectures	Anatomy, pathology
Small group discussion	Disease management
Written material	Devices, oxygen
	Travel
	Relaxation
	Coping skills
	Sexual relations
	Smoking cessation

with treatment. The best forum for this interaction is usually in a small group setting rather than a formal lecture theatre. This allows open dialogue between patient and doctor and therefore a more flexible acquisition of knowledge. Some doctors feel uncomfortable with the concept of direct confrontation with patients, fearing that the sessions may turn into open consultations. In practice, patients are hungry for knowledge about their condition and the sessions can be stimulating for doctor and patient alike.

In addition to the spoken sessions it is also valuable to reinforce them with written material in the form of a course folder or book which can be distributed at a chosen point in the course. The value of the written material lies in the ability of patients to refer to advice or reference material after the course has finished. It is also possible to include material of a sensitive nature which some patients may find difficult to discuss in public.

The remainder of this chapter will describe the content of core disease education sessions and some specific areas such as nebulizer usage, oxygen and smoking cessation. The purpose is to give readers some curriculum framework for use in their own programme.

The pathology and clinical features of chronic disabling lung disease

The majority of people who attend rehabilitation programmes in Europe and North America will be suffering from chronic airflow limitation. Most surveys suggest that about 90% of patients in the programme will come into this category. The remainder have a mixture of conditions. Some of the patients with chronic airflow limitation will have never smoked and be suffering from chronic persistent asthma, while the majority will have chronic obstructive pulmonary disease (COPD) secondary to cigarette smoking. In spite of this variety of conditions, there are similarities in the way that physical deconditioning and oppressive dyspnoea dominate the lives of patients with chronic lung disease and the benefits of multidisciplinary rehabilitation appear to be achievable in all patients with chronic respiratory disability (Foster and Thomas, 1990). In view of the overwhelming dominance of chronic airflow limitation, most of the disease education therefore relates to this condition and its management. If patients with other conditions are present during the sessions then some additional discussion can usually be contrived. The curriculum for disease education sessions should be relevant both to general medical treatment and to aims of pulmonary rehabilitation. It is therefore reasonable to place emphasis on knowledge of those factors which will alter the natural history of COPD, those factors which improve airway function, the mechanism of supportive treatment and the roles of rehabilitation and surgery (Ferguson and Cherniak, 1993).

The structure and function of the lung

The level of knowledge of pulmonary anatomy and function is likely to be overestimated even in health workers. A review of the subject is therefore a necessary prerequisite to the discussion about pathology and treatment. In particular some expansion of explanation into pathology or pathophysiology will greatly help the understanding of treatment. It is easily possible to inform patients about seemingly difficult concepts (e.g. hyperinflation and dyspnoea) if it is carefully explained and the audience is empathic.

The investigation of lung structure and function

For the purposes of rehabilitation, some description of the investigative processes of respiratory medicine is valuable. This could broadly include emphasis on radiology and pulmonary function measurements since they are relevant to diagnosis and therapy. Detailed descriptions of other procedures such as bronchoscopy may not be useful to the majority of patients.

Since the definitions of chronic bronchitis, pulmonary emphysema and COPD are epidemiological, pathological or functional, then conventional radiology is unlikely to be characteristic. However, the plain radiograph of the chest can illustrate important circumstantial evidence of chronic airflow obstruction such as hyperinflation, pulmonary hypertension and peripheral oligaemia. The use of the radiograph to diagnose emphysema with confidence is limited. By contrast, the computed tomographic (CT) scan can display the structure of the lung parenchyma with some clarity. It is possible to confirm and even quantify the presence of emphysema by CT scan. It will also delineate emphysematous bullae that may be amenable to surgery.

The measurement of lung function is a key descriptor of COPD and also an important tool to monitor progress. The basic minimum for measurement should be spirometry (forced expiratory volume in 1 s (FEV_1) and forced vital capacity (FVC)) or flow–volume curve. The peak flow measurement, which is very useful in patients with labile asthma, has little value in COPD since it does not adequately describe the nature of the airflow obstruction and may not reflect the benefits of therapy which improve either the latter or inspiratory flow rates. The FEV_1 is the most useful investigation since it is a robust measure which has been used to describe the natural history of the condition and therefore can intimate prognosis. It can also be used to stage and stratify patients with COPD. The FEV_1 declines with age at a rate of approximately 30 ml/year but this decline can rise to 150 ml/year in a susceptible smoker. Symptoms are invariably present when the FEV_1 falls below 1 l and the mortality rate of patients whose FEV_1 is less than 0.75 l is 95% over 10 years. For ease of management, a staging system based on FEV_1 has recently been proposed (American Thoracic Society, 1995).

- Stage 1: $FEV_1 > 50\%$ predicted.
- Stage 2: FEV_1 35–49% predicted.
- Stage 3: $FEV_1 < 35\%$ predicted.

Patients in stage 1 have few symptoms and are generally managed in primary care, whereas those in stages 2 and 3 generally require hospital assessment and consideration for rehabilitation and oxygen therapy. The presence of significant bronchodilator reversibility (improvement greater than 15% or 160 ml) does not necessarily imply a diagnosis of asthma but may suggest a better prognosis. In any event, the post-bronchodilator FEV_1 should be used for prognostic purposes. Although the fall of the FEV_1 below 50% predicted does have some prognostic value, it cannot predict the individual onset of disability or respiratory failure since these things may be influenced by factors other than airway calibre, such as pulmonary vascular destruction or skeletal muscle fitness. Nevertheless, it is recommended that estimation of arterial blood gases should be considered once the FEV_1 falls below 50% predicted.

In some patients more extensive tests of pulmonary function may prove valuable. For example, the plethysmographic assessment of lung volume may be helpful in patients with suspected bullous disease where the volume of trapped gas may be estimated. The measurement of carbon monoxide gas transfer helps to differentiate those patients with COPD from predominant emphysema, although this is seldom of any practical importance when it comes to rehabilitation.

The clinical features and natural history of COPD

COPD is characterized by insidious onset of progressive cough, wheeze and dyspnoea and it usually occurs in the later decades of life. The airflow obstruction is manifested by a decline in the FEV_1 which broadly mirrors the onset of symptoms, although the disease rarely comes to the attention of the physician before the FEV_1 declines to values of 50% predicted. Once airway function declines further then the risk of symptom development becomes much greater and serious disability and respiratory failure are likely once the FEV_1 falls below 35% predicted.

Cigarette smoking is the principal cause of COPD in the developed world but nevertheless only 15% of smokers will develop the condition. The risks of developing symptomatic COPD are related to age as well as past and current smoking history. In general, a smoking history of greater than 20 pack-years is necessary to make a confident diagnosis. Patients without an extensive smoking history may have chronic persistent asthma but since their airflow obstruction will not be completely reversible, they can be considered in the same manner as those with COPD. Chronic disabling symptoms from COPD usually occur towards the sixth and seventh decade of life. Patients may have little warning of impending disability since they can avoid situations which create breathlessness for some years by modifying their lifestyle. Once dyspnoea begins to interfere with daily activities there will already have been a significant reduction in pulmonary function which will be difficult to improve by medical treatment.

Dyspnoea is the cardinal symptom of chronic airflow obstruction which may be accompanied by cough and wheeze. The breathlessness is characteristically present on exertion and relieved by rest. Episodic dyspnoea which occurs at rest or at night is unlikely to be due to COPD but breathless attacks following exertion or airway irritation are common and can be treated effectively by relaxation or oxygen. Cough when present is usually productive of small to moderate quantities of mucoid sputum. As the disease progresses, other features associated with respiratory failure such as weight loss, ankle oedema or polycythaemia may become evident. In the early stages of COPD the signs on clinical examination may be confined to audible wheeze. Later on, hyperinflation and lower ribcage paradox may become evident together with alterations in the pattern of breathing and exaggerated use of the accessory muscles and shoulder girdle. Patients with extreme breathlessness may adopt unusual breathing patterns or postures to optimize mechanical or gas exchange function. Examples include pursed-lip breathing, shoulder girdle-supporting postures and reduced breathlessness on recumbency (platypnoea).

Treatment of COPD

The improvement of functional capacity by rehabilitation which includes exercise conditioning and psychosocial support is based upon the assumption that optimum medical management has already been achieved. This is usually the case when patients are referred for rehabilitation by respiratory specialists. Nevertheless, further education about the theory and practical aspects of medical treatment will improve understanding and possibly compliance. This may be particularly helpful in the areas of steroid treatment, nebulized bronchodilator use and oxygen administration where misconceptions may be present. For the purposes of teaching, the management of COPD can usefully be divided into the sections described by Ferguson and Cherniak (1993), and these aspects will be covered in the remainder of the chapter.

Altering the natural history of COPD – smoking cessation

Since cigarette smoking is the major cause of chronic disabling lung disease it makes sense to try and prevent the development of the condition or retard its development by stopping smoking. Unfortunately, the prevalence of smoking in the UK population (33%) will ensure that large numbers of the population will continue to develop lung disease. Even those who have recently given up the habit will still be vulnerable to the condition if they have quit too late. Encouraging people to give up cigarette smoking is much more difficult than persuading them not to start in the first place. It is therefore incumbent on responsible governments throughout the world to take a tough line on the sale and promotion of tobacco products. Cynically most governments take the view that the direct and indirect profits from the tobacco industry outweigh the ill health and suffering caused by disease.

The effects of smoking cessation

The effects of stopping smoking are minor but significant. Occasionally, small improvements in FEV_1 can occur as a result. Many patients also report a recurrence of productive cough as cilial function recovers. The most obvious benefits lie in the reduction of the rate of decline of FEV_1, notwithstanding that most patients will already have left it too late to preserve useful function because the onset of serious symptoms is usually delayed until airway function is severely impaired. Once cessation has occurred, the rate of decline of FEV_1 may be halved and this benefit may be seen in all ages. The more sanguine physician can, with the use of a calculator, estimate the extended prognosis obtained by stopping smoking.

Smoking cessation in practice

It is extremely difficult to persuade people to give up smoking once the habit is established. This may be stating the obvious, but it is surprising just how ineffective smoking cessation programmes can be. Even the best results can only claim prolonged abstinence rates which exceed 20% of the target population. Most smoking cessation interventions are quite correctly aimed at patients with mild or moderate impairment of lung function who have most to gain from cessation. The irony is that by the time patients are referred for pulmonary rehabilitation the majority are so severely disabled that they have actually quit smoking spontaneously but have obtained relatively little benefit from it. This raises an important point about the value of smoking cessation advice within a rehabilitation programme. When programmes contain a large proportion of severely impaired patients the inclusion of general smoking cessation advice may be inappropriate. Those patients who have quit will not like to be reminded of their folly and the few remaining smokers would benefit more properly from individual advice.

Practical smoking cessation

Given the poor expectation of success in smoking cessation programmes it is understandable that many physicians are reluctant to become involved in the process. Nevertheless, it is recognized that one of the key facilitators of a change of lifestyle is the physician's strong and ongoing commitment to encourage the smoker to stop. It is also difficult to quit if other members of the family are not supportive or continue to smoke themselves. Usually smoking cessation is carried out on an individual basis but group therapy has been explored. Whatever the environment, the potential quitter will need to prepare the process by setting up a supportive social matrix and planning how to deal with stress and possible temporary relapses. Sudden withdrawal is more likely to be associated with permanent cessation than a gradual reduction in cigarette consumption, which will always be susceptible to intercurrent lack of commitment. A seemingly successful strategy is to set a quit date with the encouragement of the physician and subsequently retain contact in person or by telephone to encourage adherence. Adherence can be checked by expired carbon monoxide monitoring or urinary cotinine measurement.

It may be helpful to view cigarette smoking as a physical as well as a social addiction in some patients with COPD. The sufferer is then seen as the victim of pharmacological incarceration rather than the perpetrator of an antisocial habit. For this reason nicotine substitutes may be seen as a useful adjunct to individual or group therapy. The physical side-effects of withdrawal which occur immediately after quitting can be ameliorated by nicotine replacement in those patients who appear physically addicted. Both nicotine chewing gum and nicotine patches have been shown to be effective in placebo-controlled trials. As expected, nicotine replacement is more effective in the context of a structured cessation

Tips for smoking cessation

Agree a quit date

Provide strong medical endorsement

Recruit family support

Consider nicotine replacement

View smoker as victim

Long-term support is needed

Box 8.2

programme. The ideal duration of replacement therapy is unknown but may be in the region of 6–8 weeks. Nicotine replacement therapy is not available on National Health Service prescription in the UK.

There are other routes to smoking cessation which may be valuable to some smokers. There are a number of commercial programmes which include group therapy, telephone support and education which claim reasonable success rates. Acupuncture and hypnosis have also been promoted as quitting adjuncts. In all these examples the financial commitment may be an important stimulus. Overall the most important predictor of success may be individual motivation from whatever direction.

Medical treatment for COPD – improving airway function

The initial treatment of symptomatic COPD begins with encouragement to stop smoking, followed by efforts to reverse airflow obstruction. In the first instance this will involve the prescription of inhaled or oral bronchodilator and consideration of inhaled steroid. The treatment of acute exacerbations may require oral corticosteroids and antibiotics.

Bronchodilators

Bronchodilator drugs are the mainstay of pharmacological palliation for COPD. As in asthma, the greater understanding that the patient has of the mechanism of action and mode of delivery of drugs, the more likely there is to be compliance and effectiveness. Therefore there should be as much emphasis on education and training in COPD as there is in the management of asthma. There are, however, important general differences in the mode of action and the spectrum of use of bronchodilators in COPD which are worth describing (Table 8.2). The most important distinction lies in the value of demonstrating bronchodilator reversibility as

Table 8.2 Bronchodilator drugs in chronic obstructive pulmonary disease

	Route	Unwanted effects
β-agonists		
Salbutamol	Inhaled	Tremor
Terbutaline		Cramps
Anticholinergic		
Ipratropium	Inhaled	Dry mouth
Oxitropium		Glaucoma
		Prostatism
Theophyllines		
Aminophylline	Oral	Gastrointestinal intolerance
Theophylline		Drug interactions, arrhythmias

a presumption of effective treatment. Bronchodilator reversibility can only be demonstrated in a minority of patients with COPD as compared to asthma.

Although it is frequently requested by clinicians, the value of demonstrating bronchodilator reversibility does not accurately predict the treatment response. Obviously if it is present, the demonstration of bronchodilator response is likely to be associated with a clinical improvement with treatment. However, the absence of a significant measured response is often associated with a subjective improvement. The absence of significant bronchodilator response should not be used to deny such treatment to patients if they find the drug symptomatically beneficial. The main reason for this apparent discrepancy lies in the subtlety with which bronchodilators may have their effect. In COPD the effect of bronchodilatation may be to improve airway calibre expressed as FEV_1, but may also improve lung mechanics by improving inspiratory flow or by reduction of hyperinflation or the work of breathing. The objective confirmation of bronchodilator action may require the measurement of exercise performance or dyspnoea or even quality of life questionnaire.

As in asthma, β-agonist drugs are the bronchodilators of choice but by a much smaller margin. β-Agonists are relatively less effective in COPD, whilst anticholinergic drugs may be more effective. The principles of bronchodilator treatment in COPD suggest that more than one agent may be effective and that the doses required are usually in excess of those required in asthma and therefore more attention must be paid to unwanted effects.

β-Agonist treatment

The inhaled route for treatment is preferred in COPD and asthma since oral preparations of β-agonists have troublesome side-effects which may be even more pronounced in the older population. These include tremor and palpitations amongst others. The delivery device is largely a matter of choice and ability to comply. Many elderly patients have difficulty with inhalers and therefore a metered dose inhaler and large volume spacer is a good starting point while adequate inhaler training is obligatory. The best device is the one that suits the patient best. In mild COPD, short-acting bronchodilators (salbutamol, terbutaline) can be taken on demand or prior to exertion. As the disease progresses, larger doses (400–800 µg) may become useful and can be taken regularly. There is no evidence that the regular use of β-agonists is detrimental in COPD. The role of long-acting β-agonist drugs (salmeterol, formoterol) is not yet defined in COPD.

Anticholinergic bronchodilators

These drugs appear to be more effective in COPD than in asthma by reducing bronchomotor tone. There is therefore some rationale for having a lower threshold for their introduction, particularly since they appear to have a longer duration of action than β-agonists. The debate about whether β-agonists and anticholinergic drugs are synergistic in action has waxed and waned. However, it is likely that moderate doses of both drugs can achieve maximal bronchodilatation while trading off the side-effects of each.

Theophyllines

The use of oral sustained-release theophylline has a historical prominence in the management of COPD. Its use appears to be a matter of individual or cultural choice. Theophyllines are not as effective as they can be in asthma and their use can be complicated by troublesome side-effects which necessitate the measurement of blood levels. Further complications may also ensue by interaction with some common drugs including erythromycin and cimetidine which may inadvertently increase the blood levels to within the toxic range. The drugs have some theoretical advantages in COPD on respiratory muscle or cardiac function but these are often outweighed by their inconvenience of use. It is usual, in the UK at least, to introduce theophyllines as a trial only when treatment with β-agonists and anticholinergic drugs has proved inadequate.

Nebulized bronchodilator drugs

Patients who are admitted to hospital with an exacerbation of COPD often attribute their recovery to the use of nebulized bronchodilator drugs. This is understandable since nebulizers are invariably used in this circumstance. However, there are many other factors which participate in the improvement. These include antibiotics, oral corticosteroids, oxygen, nursing care and sanctuary. Nevertheless there is now a public perception that home nebulized bronchodilator treatment is appropriate for moderate to severe grades of COPD. The advantages of nebulized treatment include the ability to deliver big doses of β-agonist and anticholinergic bronchodilators in a form which can be rapidly and easily administered. The disadvantage of nebulized treatment is that it can overshadow other equally important aspects of treatment and expose the patient to greater risk of unwanted effects. The other prejudice against nebulized treatment is that it is often no more effective than correctly taken inhaler therapy and carries with it a considerable increase in annual prescribing costs which may exceed £2000 per annum.

In spite of these caveats, many patients do gain substantial relief from home nebulizers and should be able to obtain them if required. Provision of domiciliary apparatus varies widely throughout the country and there is also no clear consensus as to which patients should benefit. However, British Thoracic Society guidelines on the subject are planned. For the interim there are some guidelines for assessment and some responsibilities for providers which should be followed.

Like bronchodilator reversibility, the assessments may need to be quite subtle to confirm the subjective response. There is also little consensus as to how the nebulized drugs should be used once they are prescribed. They can be used on demand for breathless episodes as with asthma or used on a regular basis up to four times per day.

Corticosteroid treatment

In contrast to asthma, the role of corticosteroid treatment is less clear in COPD. It is usually highly relevant to patients with other conditions where prolonged oral corticosteroid treatment may take a prominent role in the management. Since there is a high level of public anxiety about steroid treatment in general, it is one of the most important educational issues in a rehabilitation programme.

With respect to COPD, there is increasing evidence that inflammation may have a subsidiary role in the pathogenesis of the condition, though the size of that role and its potential correction by steroid treatment are unknown. It is also important to remember that older patients may be more susceptible to the side-effects of treatment. Current thinking sug-

Guide for the issue of compressors and nebulizers

Prior review by appropriate specialist

Ensure correct use of current inhalers

Therapeutic trial with appropriate outcome measures

Clear demonstration of use

Written instructions with issue

Service and repair arrangements

Loan service for breakdown and holiday

Box 8.3

gests that oral corticosteroids may have a place in two areas of management: first as a therapeutic trial and second as treatment in the acute exacerbation.

Trials of oral steroid

A prolonged trial of prednisolone in stable COPD (30 mg for 2 weeks) will produce a significant improvement in FEV_1 in approximately 20% of patients (Postma and Renkema, 1995). This subset may also be identified by bronchodilator reversibility. These patients may have a better prognosis which is determined by the post-steroid or bronchodilator FEV_1. It is important to identify this subgroup which may benefit from a treatment approach similar to that of asthma which may include inhaled or prolonged oral corticosteroids. Although the evidence for this effect is not yet available, it is reasonable to suppose that it might be true.

The other circumstance in which oral steroid treatment is used is the acute exacerbation. These are usually treated with antibiotics, increased bronchodilators and oral prednisolone. In these circumstances the short course of treatment seems to be effective but should not be prolonged beyond recovery.

Inhaled corticosteroid treatment in COPD

The widespread use of inhaled corticosteroid drugs in asthma has carried over to patients with COPD without any concrete justification for their use. Large numbers of patients are currently taking this medication with the attendant costs and risks. There are presently at least two large multicentre trials under way (Isolde and Euroscop) which will answer the question as to whether inhaled corticosteroids will reduce the rate of decline of FEV_1 in COPD. For the moment it is probably worth consid-

225

ering the introduction of inhaled corticosteroids in patients who demonstrate a significant steroid or bronchodilator response. The same qualifications apply to the delivery of inhaled steroids in COPD with regard to education and inhaler devices as in asthma. There appears to be no role for anti-inflammatory agents other than inhaled steroids in COPD.

Antibiotics

An explanation of the correct use of antibiotics is helpful since patients often receive them in a variety of circumstances. Antibiotics are invaluable in the treatment of pneumonia but their role in the management of acute exacerbation of COPD is less clear. Many exacerbations are not due directly to bacterial lower respiratory tract infections and antibiotic treatment may not be required. A guide as to whether antibiotics are necessary may be judged clinically by the presence of coloured sputum, fever, chest signs, leucocytosis or radiological change.

The other area where antibiotics have an important role is in bronchiectasis. Here a careful explanation of the distinction between colonization and infection is required. Signs of intercurrent infection include increased sputum volume, darker colour or haemoptysis or features of systemic upset. In some cases regular intravenous antibiotics or prolonged oral administration is recommended while some patients take daily nebulized antibiotic.

Other drugs in respiratory medicine

Most other drugs in respiratory medicine are used for short-term treatment or in rather specialized circumstances and do not usually become topics of discussion in the rehabilitation groups. Occasionally the questions do touch on some aspects which require answers. Examples include mucolytic drugs which generally have no useful role, though they are presently being re-examined. Other examples which generate enquiry are sedatives and stimulant drugs. There appears to be a limited place for some opioid or sedative medication like codeine in the amelioration of distressing dyspnoea. There is a similarly small place for respiratory stimulant drugs such as progesterone or acetazolamide in chronic, and doxapram or aminophylline in acute respiratory failure.

Supportive therapy – oxygen treatment

There is a perception amongst health professionals and the public that oxygen treatment is the last and most desperate therapeutic manoeuvre for patients in respiratory failure. Very few health care professionals are

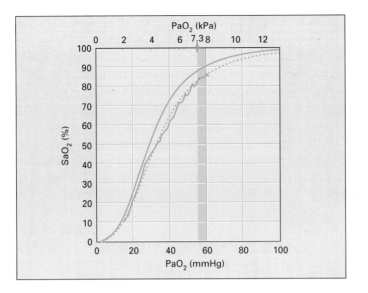

Fig. 8.1 The shape of the oxygen dissociation curve (oxygen saturation (Sao_2) versus partial pressure (Pao_2)) determines that oxygen delivery, which is dependent upon saturation, will only be assured if the Pao_2 exceeds 8 kPa. Modified from Calverley and Pride (1995), with permission.

familiar with the various indications for oxygen treatment or with the methods of delivery. It is not necessary for patients to be on established respiratory failure to benefit, nor is it necessary for them to have irreversible disease to qualify for treatment.

Tissue oxygen delivery and respiratory failure

By qualitative definition, respiratory failure is described as inadequate tissue oxygen supply. Of course, the lungs are only one element in the chain which links the external environment to the cellular oxygen requirement. Inadequate oxygen supply can occur if the environmental supply of oxygen is inadequate, as it is at high altitude, and it can also occur if there is inadequate cardiac output or haemoglobin to transport oxygen to the tissues. However, for the purposes of education to rehabilitation groups it is reasonable to assume that these factors are not operating and that the damaged lung is the cause of failure.

The formal definition of respiratory failure (at sea level) is set by blood gas tensions of a partial pressure of arterial oxygen (Pao_2) <7.3 kPa with or without an elevated partial pressure of arterial carbon dioxide ($Paco_2$; >6.5 kPa). The reason for this precision is the shape of the oxygen dissociation curve for haemoglobin which determines the amount of oxygen which can bind to haemoglobin and be available for delivery to the tissues (Fig. 8.1). A value of blood gas oxygen tension above 7.3 kPa is therefore associated with nearly normal oxygen saturation of haemoglobin and adequate oxygen delivery is assured under normal conditions.

However, under conditions of exercise, sleep, illness or altitude these certainties need not apply. It is therefore not sensible to consider respiratory failure as a static event, but one which is more likely to occur in patients with lung disease given the prevailing circumstances. The principles of management of respiratory failure and oxygen treatment are common to all types of lung disease which result in hypoxia but as usual, patients with COPD will make up the majority. As a principle, an educational discussion about oxygen therapy should attempt to demystify a subject which is associated with terminal illness and intimidating pulmonary physiology.

Methods of oxygen supply and delivery

Non-atmospheric oxygen is available in three forms: compressed gas, liquid oxygen and the oxygen concentrator (Table 8.3). In the future other systems such as the oxygen separator may become available. Hospital supplies in the UK are usually liquid oxygen while home supplies are in cylinder or oxygen concentrator form depending upon the amount of oxygen that is required. In other countries liquid oxygen may be the domestic system of choice. Liquid oxygen and cylinders are supplied by the gas company. Cylinders may be prescribed in various sizes to the patient and delivered to the patient via the pharmacist. By contrast, oxygen concentrators are devices which are installed in the home and generate oxygen-rich air by absorption of nitrogen as it passes over a column of xeolyte crystals. They are powered by electricity and the cost of this can be reimbursed to the patient.

The delivery of supplementary oxygen to the conscious patient is achieved through one of three routes: face mask, nasal cannula and occasionally transtracheal cannula. The face mask with a Venturi system of entrainment provides the most accurate fractional concentration of

Table 8.3 Suitability of types of oxygen source			
	Cylinder	*Oxygen concentrator*	*Liquid oxygen*
Short burst	+	–	–
Long-term oxygen therapy	–	+	+
Ambulatory	+	–	+
Portable	+	–	+

inspired oxygen (Fio_2) and allows higher fractions of oxygen to be used. The nasal cannulae supply a small flow of oxygen more discretely for entrainment but are less accurate in their delivery, though under most conditions this is unimportant. A flow rate of 1 l/min usually relates to an Fio_2 of approximately 0.24 and 2 l to 0.28. Humidification is not usually required for these methods of oxygen delivery at flow rates below 5 l/min. Transtracheal oxygen delivery is more popular in North America than in the UK. The technique involves the surgical placement of a permanent catheter in the trachea. This allows very low flow rates of oxygen to be used in the most cosmetically acceptable fashion. The disadvantages relate to the possible need for humidification and a tendency for mucus obstruction of the cannula.

The efficiency of all types of delivery device can be increased by devices which limit the flow of oxygen to inspiration only. The two forms of oxygen-conserving device which are available are the reservoir cannula and the demand-pulse valve. The former stores the continuous oxygen supply in a reservoir for use in inspiration. The latter triggers a pulse of oxygen at the beginning of inspiration. In practice these devices only have value where oxygen supply is at a premium, as for example with ambulatory or airline oxygen supplies.

Symptomatic (short-burst) oxygen treatment

For people who are breathless with lung disease the presence of an oxygen cylinder at home can provide comfort and relief. Symptomatic oxygen can relieve episodic dyspnoea brought on by exacerbation, exercise and emotion. Even if patients have been shown to have a Pao_2 above the threshold definition of 7.3 kPa in the laboratory, they may still suffer from episodic hypoxia under some domestic conditions which can be relieved by oxygen administration. Although in this regard the prescriber should be aware of the theoretical worsening of hypercapnia by oxygen treatment, this is most unlikely in patients with a normal $Paco_2$ and the respiratory drive characteristic of 'pink puffer' type patients who complain of dyspnoea. Even if the cylinder is never used, it can provide a source of confidence for a patient to weather a storm and stay out of hospital. It can therefore be a very cost-effective placebo.

Long-term oxygen therapy (LTOT)

In patients with COPD and demonstrable hypoxaemia, prolonged treatment with oxygen in excess of 15 h/day has been shown to improve survival and reduce pulmonary hypertension. It may also improve the poor health-related quality of life perceived by these patients but is unlikely

Box 8.4

Guidelines for long-term oxygen therapy

COPD with FEV_1 <1.5 l

Cor pulmonale

Pao_2 <7.3 kPa + $Paco_2$ >6.5 kPa

Stability over 3 weeks

COPD = Chronic obstructive pulmonary disease; FEV_1 = forced expiratory volume in 1 s; Pao_2 = partial pressure of arterial oxygen; $Paco_2$ = partial pressure of arterial carbon dioxide.

to reverse their social isolation. This practice originates from the results of two large clinical trials performed almost 20 years ago in the UK and in North America which have not so far been repeated (Nocturnal Oxygen Therapy Trial Group, 1980; Medical Research Council, 1981). The prescription of LTOT in the UK can only be considered after careful physiological assessment in a patient on optimum treatment during a period of clinical stability.

Since the assessment requires the repeated measurement of blood gases, it usually has to be performed at a hospital. In the UK the assessment responsibility lies with the hospital physician and the prescribing responsibility lies with the general practitioner. This is an unsatisfactory situation which leads to inappropriate, unassessed or omitted prescriptions. In Scotland the hospital physician has both the assessment and prescribing responsibility.

Once a prescription for LTOT has been issued, it is usually provided by installation of a domiciliary oxygen concentrator, or in a few areas liquid oxygen. The oxygen concentrator is installed in a convenient place in the home with sufficient flexible tubing to cover the living and sleeping areas. The flow rate prescription (up to 4 l/min) is determined in the laboratory by the flow rate necessary to achieve a Pao_2 >8.0 kPa or oxygen saturation by pulse oximetry (Spo_2) >90% without significant rise in $Paco_2$. The flow rate may need to be adjusted upwards for increased activity and downwards for sleep. Once installed, it is important to remember that circumstances can change and the prescription has to be reviewed regularly for compliance and accuracy. This often means a visit to hospital which can be avoided if a respiratory nurse is available to visit.

Portable and ambulatory oxygen

Patients requiring LTOT should not be under 'house arrest' during their treatment. Both portable oxygen supplies and ambulatory devices are available to cover activities outside the home. Portable oxygen cylinders which can be prescribed on the drug tariff (PD size) are small enough to be carried by a carer to accompany car journeys or short absences from base. Obviously these can be useful, but they are too heavy for the patient to carry to increase their own work rate and independence. Ambulatory oxygen devices are carried by the patient and supply additional oxygen for exercise. The most common variety is the light-weight portable cylinder, made of aluminium or carbon fibre, which is filled from a larger reservoir cylinder in the home. They cannot be filled from an oxygen concentrator.

If liquid oxygen is the domiciliary source then it can be decanted to a small pack for ambulatory use. The endurance of these devices varies considerably, from less than 1 h to 12 h. Obviously, the very short-range devices are self-defeating and all of the techniques are enhanced by the addition of oxygen-conserving devices. In the committed patient, the most successful method appears to be the combination of transtracheal cannula and liquid oxygen.

There is no agreement about physiological assessment for patients requiring ambulatory oxygen apart from the demonstration of exercise-induced hypoxaemia. In the UK there is no National Health Service provision for ambulatory oxygen devices, though some respiratory units may have some to loan or use during rehabilitation programmes.

Air travel and respiratory disease

Today, many people with lung disease and even respiratory failure travel by air without mishap. Many airlines cater for patients with lung disease who require oxygen, and questions about air travel are one of the commonest forms of enquiry to Breathe Easy. In spite of the increasing popularity of air travel, the advice which patients receive is often unclear or incomplete. Modern commercial airplanes have cabins which are pressurized to 1500–2500 m (5000–8000 ft) depending upon the type of plane. Patients with lung disease are therefore exposed to several increased risks which would not be present on the ground. First, there is a risk that the slight rarification of the atmosphere on ascent may lead to rupture of a portion of the lung which was not able to empty rapidly. Such risk of lung rupture or pneumothorax is very small during normal flight, except perhaps where there is already a pre-existing pneumothorax or bulla. In addition, if the aircraft were to suffer an accidental decompression at cruising altitude, the serious loss of pressure would affect the sufferer with lung disease first. Hopefully this situation is extremely rare.

The second issue relates to the fall in partial pressure of oxygen in the cabin atmosphere which may make already hypoxic patients worse. In practice, it appears that if patients with COPD are in borderline respiratory failure they will be able to adapt to the environment for short periods of flight. This can be assessed at ground level by a hypoxic simulation test, in a lung function laboratory. If patients need oxygen on the ground then they will require it in flight.

Aircraft do not carry sufficient regular supplies for continuous use and if people need to use supplementary oxygen they have to bring it with them in the form of cylinders. This has to be organized in advance with the airline and a charge is usually made.

People with lung disease are also susceptible to the other hazards of air travel. These include the dry atmosphere which may thicken bronchial secretions and the lack of mobility which favours the development of thromboembolism. Standard advice to all travellers should be to avoid dehydration and be as mobile as possible during the flight.

Non-invasive ventilatory support

The prognosis for some patients with chronic ventilatory failure has altered dramatically with the development of techniques for the non-invasive support of ventilation (Simonds and Elliot, 1995). Strictly, this falls into the category of medical treatment rather than rehabilitation and will not be described in excessive detail. Nevertheless, patients who are receiving such support will attend rehabilitation programmes and discussion of the techniques forms a natural topic for education.

We are familiar with the concept of artificial support of ventilation for patients with acute respiratory failure on intensive care units. This normally takes the form of tracheal intubation and intermittent positive-pressure ventilation (IPPV). The last decade has seen the re-exploration of previously discarded methods of ventilatory support for the management of chronic ventilatory failure. The most suitable patients for this type of therapy are those with disorders of the respiratory muscles or bony ribcage which lead to hypercapnic respiratory failure, which usually first becomes evident at night. A typical example of a suitable patient would be one with a paralytic scoliosis due to polio who gradually develops morning headache, daytime somnolence and cor pulmonale some decades after the original illness. Other examples include those with congenital scoliosis, thoracoplasty and other causes of respiratory muscle weakness. More controversially, the techniques have recently been investigated for patients with COPD in both acute and chronic phases of respiratory failure (Wedzicha and Meecham Jones, 1996).

There are several devices which are available for the non-invasive support of ventilation. Initially, negative pressure devices such as the tank ventilator (iron lung) or cuirass respirators were used. Although these are effective, they are relatively expensive and can provoke upper-airway obstruction in some patients. The alternative popular approach is to apply intermittent positive pressure to the airway via the nose or mouth. This has been made possible by the development of silicone masks for continuous positive airways pressure which can also be used for nasal IPPV (NIPPV). These masks can provide a comfortable seal which allows a small bedside ventilator to inflate the lungs with relatively little air leak. There are now a wide variety of inexpensive ventilators suitable for the purpose which vary in complexity. Some machines are derivatives of the conventional intensive therapy unit ventilator, while others provide ventilation with simple bilevel pressure support. Usually, NIPPV is only necessary during the night to correct and reverse ventilatory failure and the progress of treatment can be monitored intermittently by sleep studies of oxygen saturation and transcutaneous carbon dioxide.

The success of this form of treatment is most evident in those patients with chronic respiratory muscle weakness or scoliosis. The prognosis for this group has changed from a dismal expectation of a premature death to a nearly normal life expectancy. In other cases, particularly those with progressive neuromuscular disorders, the ventilatory support does not prolong life but does improve the quality and reduce the anxiety of carers. In patients with COPD there is not yet any clear recommendation for the application of non-invasive ventilatory support. It appears that, in skilful hands, NIPPV may be helpful in the management of acute respiratory failure in the hospital ward setting and therefore avoid intensive therapy unit admissions. The benefit of long-term, nocturnal domiciliary NIPPV in patients with COPD has not yet been determined.

It is necessary to get this important therapeutic development in perspective since it is obviously extremely important to those selected patients with appropriate conditions who will have dramatic improvements in prognosis and quality of life. However, this is only likely to apply to approximately 1500 patients in the UK on the present indications and a minority of those who attend rehabilitation programmes.

The intense medical interest in the future of NIPPV should be balanced with a recognition of the nature of the market for rehabilitation.

Surgery and lung disease

Patients with chronic lung disease are interested in the effects of surgery for two major reasons. First, those patients attending rehabilitation programmes will be of an age where incidental illnesses requiring surgery may be necessary and they are often disadvantaged or disqualified by virtue of their respiratory impairment. Second, there is renewed interest in surgery as a form of active treatment for pulmonary emphysema.

Anaesthesia and surgery for patients with lung disease

Anaesthesia and surgery for any indication carry a risk of death or complication which will be increased in patients with chronic lung disease. Broadly this risk will be related to the degree of pulmonary impairment but can be increased by continued cigarette smoking or sputum production. The disadvantages of general anaesthesia can be offset by the judicious use of local or regional techniques. It is often difficult for the physician who is supervising a rehabilitation programme to give specific advice about the risks and conduct of anaesthesia other than to outline the general principles. Where there is a demand for knowledge about this subject it may be necessary to invite an anaesthetist to talk to the group on the risks and conduct of anaesthesia. This is more likely to be practical in the wider setting of the Breathe Easy support groups rather than the intimacy of the small groups in the rehabilitation programmes.

Thoracic surgery rarely improves lung function except in a few specific circumstances. Most thoracic surgery either removes lung tissue or temporarily damages the lung so that there is an immediate reduction in lung function to which the patient must adapt and recover. This applies to procedures such as lobectomy or pneumonectomy as well as thoracotomies which do not involve lung resection. More optimistically, there are a few thoracic surgical procedures which actually improve lung function. Decortication of the lung is one operation which can correct the late effects of pyogenic or tuberculous empyema up to 20 years after the illness and should therefore always be considered. The other area where surgery might be effective is in carefully selected patients with pulmonary emphysema.

Thoracic surgery for emphysema

Surgery for pulmonary emphysema has always been recognized to be successful in patients with bullous disease (Morgan, 1995). These patients often have excessive dyspnoea which is associated with hyperinflation. The bulla may be visible on a plain chest radiograph but can be characterized in more detail by CT. The indications for surgery may simply be the presence of symptoms and the identification of a reasonable-sized bulla on CT. The details of the surgery may vary but include formal thoracotomy and bullectomy or the less invasive approach of intracavitary drainage and, more recently, video-assisted thoracoscopic techniques. The results of this type of surgery are excellent, with immediate improvements in lung function and reduction in symptoms which may be sustained for many years.

The most recent developments in the surgical management have been the rediscovery of the possible benefits of pulmonary reconstruction in more generalized emphysema. In theory, the reduction of lung volume by surgery may improve the symptoms of dyspnoea in selected cases where hyperinflation is the major pathophysiological feature. This type of surgery has been explored in the past but the technical demands of the surgery and the lack of precision of preoperative investigation have hampered development. In recent years the development of more air-tight stapling devices and improvements in imaging by CT have allowed this area to be revisited (Cooper *et al.*, 1995; Sciurba *et al.*, 1996). In selected patients, it appears that excision of approximately one-third of the most emphysematous areas of both lungs can be associated with improvement of both lung function and quality of life. The actual mechanism for the improvement in FEV_1 that is observed may be difficult to understand but is probably related to the recovery of elastic recoil in the remaining lung. It further appears as if pulmonary rehabilitation is an obligatory prerequisite to the success of surgery by preconditioning the patients prior to operation.

For the present, the long-term results of volume reduction surgery have not been evaluated, and widespread introduction of the procedure cannot yet be recommended. However, this is potentially a very exciting development which may be able to help selected patients with COPD on a large scale and also increase the demand and indications for pulmonary rehabilitation.

References

American Thoracic Society. (1995) Standards for the diagnosis and care of patients with chronic obstructive pulmonary disease. *Am. J. Respir. Crit. Care Med.* **152**:s77–120.

Calverley, P.M.A., and Pride, N.B. (eds) (1995) *Chronic Obstructive Lung Disease.* London: Chapman & Hall, p. 505.

Cooper, J.D., Trulock, E.P., Triantafillou, A.N. *et al.* (1995) Bilateral pneumectomy (volume reduction) for chronic obstructive pulmonary disease. *J. Thorac. Cardiovasc. Surg.* **109**:106–19.

Ferguson, G.T., and Cherniak, R.M. (1993) Management of chronic obstructive pulmonary disease. *N. Engl. J. Med.* **328**:1017–22.

Foster, S., and Thomas, H.M. (1990) Pulmonary rehabilitation in lung disease other than chronic obstructive pulmonary disease. *Am. Rev. Respir. Dis.* **141**:601–4.

Medical Research Council Working Party. (1981) Long term domiciliary oxygen therapy in chronic hypoxic cor pulmonale complicating chronic bronchitis and emphysema. *Lancet* **i**:681–6.

Disease education and medical support

Morgan, M.D.L. (1995) Bullous lung disease. In: *Chronic Obstructive Lung Disease* (eds P.M.A. Calverley and N.B. Pride). London: Chapman & Hall, pp. 547–59.

Nocturnal Oxygen Therapy Trial Group. (1980) Continuous or nocturnal oxygen therapy in chronic hypoxemic chronic obstructive lung disease. *Ann. Intern. Med.* **102**:29–36.

Postma, D.S., and Renkema, T.E.J. (1995) Corticosteroid treatment. In: *Chronic Obstructive Lung Disease* (eds P.M.A. Calverley and N.B. Pride). London: Chapman & Hall, pp. 448–59.

Sciurba, F.C., Rogers, R.M., Keenan, R.J. *et al.* (1996) Improvement in pulmonary function and elastic recoil after lung-reduction surgery for diffuse emphysema. *N. Engl. J. Med.* **334**:1095–9.

Simonds, A.K., and Elliot, M.W. (1995) Outcome of domiciliary nasal intermittent positive pressure ventilation in restrictive and obstructive disorders. *Thorax* **50**:604–9.

Toshima, M.T., Kaplan, R.M., and Ries, A.L. (1990) Experimental evaluation of rehabilitation in chronic obstructive pulmonary disease: short term effects on exercise endurance and health status. *Health Psychol.* **9**:237–52.

Wedzicha, J.A., and Meecham Jones, D.J. (1996) Domiciliary ventilation in chronic obstructive pulmonary disease: where are we? *Thorax* **51**:455–57.

9. The role of the respiratory nurse and home care

A. Heslop

Former Respiratory Nurse, Department of Medicine, Charing Cross Hospital, London

Practical Pulmonary Rehabilitation.
Edited by Mike Morgan and Sally Singh.
Published in 1997 by Chapman & Hall, London.
ISBN 0 412 61810 9.

Introduction

This chapter will discuss the potential role of a respiratory nurse in the UK today within educational and professional constraints. It will also suggest how nurses can use rehabilitation concepts in their practice and offers practical ideas and methods that may benefit patients limited by breathlessness in their everyday lives, whether in hospital or at home.

Nursing – professional and educational issues

Nichols (1980) suggests that rehabilitation is the appropriate term to embrace many physical, social and organizational aspects of patient aftercare that require more than acute short-term definitive care. Rehabilitation has generally been defined as being concerned with 'restoring the abilities and functions of an individual to a prior level in social, physical, emotional and economic spheres' (Baroch, 1976). What role do nurses play in this field? Until relatively recently, nurses learnt about the practice of nursing and patients' experience of illness within a hospital setting. For this reason, nurses may have been adequately prepared to deal with acute short-term illness. Whilst the literature suggests that nurses do have a role in rehabilitation (Myco, 1986), it is believed that they have less clarity about what that role is.

There are several issues here pertinent to nursing and how the parameters of nursing functions may have been translated into practice. Traditionally, nurses organized their work around a series of tasks that had been deemed necessary. How this work was achieved was frequently determined by the routines and time constraints of the institution, using task allocation as a method of nursing work to organize care delivery. This enabled supervisor nurses to control the nursing work of largely unqualified, continually changing workers (Proctor, 1989). However, as suggested by Miller (1985), the organization system of care has contributed to a patient being a passive recipient and being increasingly dependent in the recovery process. Furthermore, this method did not enable nurses to acquaint themselves with their patients and served to create an emotional distance between nurses and patients (Menzies, 1960). This discouraged nurses from learning about patients' individual needs and their capacities of daily living activities. Relevant skills, such as assessing and teaching patients, were not recognized as important or a necessary component of preparing patients for discharge. Medical care, whilst including rehabilitation, has taken a functional approach and formerly nurse educational curricula were shaped by medical diagnosis. There has been a focus on curing the problem, neglecting the experience of illness and the emotions incurred in loss of health and its consequences to patient and family.

During the past decade the UK Central Council's proposals to reform preregistration nursing education, often referred to as Project 2000, have been introduced (Emerton, 1986). This also places nurse education into a higher educational framework, involving educational placements in both institutional and community settings. The curriculum is more health-(as opposed to disease-)related. Underlying this need for radical change in nurse education is poor recruitment, emphasis on cost-effectiveness and value for money, as well as government policy shifts towards the community provision of care and emphasis on the prevention of ill health.

In the future nursing may be better prepared to play a more defined role in the rehabilitation process. However, this will also be subject to attention being drawn to the needs of the chronically ill before rehabilitation achieves status and profile in nurse education (Gibbon, 1992).

The role of the respiratory nurse

The role of the respiratory nurse is new but does have historical roots in the tuberculosis family visitor (Ministry of Health and Ministry of Education, 1965). As tuberculosis began to decrease, some nurses assumed responsibility for other activities. Respiratory nursing has arguably derived its practice from delegated medical tasks, such as nebulization of medicine and oxygen therapy. Respiratory nurses will certainly need to work closely with doctors along the lines of the medical model with patients who are severely ill, but they also need to identify models of respiratory care which distinguish between, but include, both health and social care (Heslop, 1993).

Increasingly, nurses have been appointed to become respiratory nurses within respiratory medical teams, are usually hospital based and may include home visiting. The role and functions vary and may be initiated by a respiratory consultant. Two evaluations of nurse interventions (Cockcroft *et al.*, 1987; Littlejohn *et al.*, 1991), initiated by the Royal College of Physicians report in 1981 on disabling chest disease, have in part spurred on the nursing role in the expanding specialty of respiratory medicine. Respiratory nurses may continue to update their knowledge through conferences and there is now a respiratory nursing course available as a forum for this specialism within the Royal College of Nursing.

Chronic lung disease may begin at an early age and it is a slow and progressive disease. People often tolerate symptoms for a long time before seeking medical treatment (Zola, 1973). Communication of information is perhaps the most important aspect of care when diagnosis is confirmed (Locker, 1983). Nurses can be teachers in the early stages of this illness, assisting people in preventing health deterioration and later in providing rehabilitation strategies.

Rehabilitation

Rehabilitation usually concerns the care of patients with long-term, and frequently permanent illness. This chapter discusses the care of patients who cannot be cured of respiratory ill health and therefore the aim is to limit disease progression and minimize symptoms and function limitation (Lertzman and Cherniak, 1976). Programmes may involve several different approaches, including medical, psychological, physical and educational, to assist patients in becoming fitter and better informed about their health and hopefully to be more in control of their lives.

Respiratory nursing in practice

The nursing and advisory role of the respiratory nurse concerning pulmonary rehabilitation will be briefly explored as relevant to the hospital setting. Discharge preparation and home care will be discussed in detail.

The respiratory nurse is required to work effectively within a large multidisciplinary team where collaboration is essential to provide comprehensive care. The respiratory nurse may be an adviser and teacher, working within a respiratory medical team, who receives referrals and may follow up patients at home or may be the ward sister in this field. There are different interpretations of this role, although increasingly a respiratory nurse specialist is employed within a respiratory specialty.

Pulmonary rehabilitation, discussed here, is considered as a necessary approach to assist patients to re-establish independence and go home better prepared. The nursing care which is outlined concerns principles for devising planned care that is responsive to the limitations imposed on the patient by the experience of breathlessness, recognizing that this will have a psychosocial impact on the individual's life and family. This may be short-term, for example, a young person with pneumonia or a person with chronic bronchitis admitted into hospital with an acute exacerbation. There is an inadequate knowledge base to evaluate which nursing interventions benefit breathless patients. However, it is valuable to have nurses who are experienced and sensitive to the needs of breathless patients to support nursing practice. The approach to nursing breathless patients is discussed in three sections, commencing with the patient in hospital, preparing for discharge and continuing rehabilitation at home.

The breathless patient in hospital

Skilled care and comfort underpin the approach to nursing a patient who is breathless. The assessment process is best accomplished by a nurse being present and observing the patient whilst assisting him or her to be physically safe and comfortable. On admission, some information is usually available to begin nursing the breathless patient. Therefore nursing principles may be thought of in three interlinked areas:

- The therapeutic plan.
- Nursing care.
- Communication.

The nurse has responsibilities to coordinate and carry out the therapeutic plan so that the patient receives prescribed medical care and changes in clinical status are observed and reported. This will invariably require recording physiological data. The therapeutic plan will be best served if nursing care is founded on interpersonal qualities that convey professional competence and concerned care to the patient.

This is illustrated by an example: a patient arriving with distressing breathlessness will receive medicines utilizing various methods of delivery. This aspect of care is a priority but may well cause initial distress, for example wearing an oxygen mask. Therefore these treatments should be accompanied by simple explanations. This helps the patient feel included and involved.

The patient is positioned in bed or a chair so that breathlessness is minimized and he or she feels physically supported to receive supervised treatment. Simple measures, such as lengthening the oxygen tubing to accommodate a range of mobility, a contact bell to summon help and nutritious drinks nearby, aid recovery and will promote independence. Elderly people often have lower back pain, may well be thin and have different body shapes such as barrel chest or kyphosis of the spine. These factors and the associated breathlessness causing potential lack of oxygen are indicators for calculating pressure risk (Waterlow, 1985) as part of early assessment to prevent soreness or skin breakdown. Arranging pillows and bedding to facilitate freedom of movement and adopting a comfortable upright position assists breathing by using accessory muscles. This also encourages expectoration of phlegm and muscle movement and enables the patient to communicate needs. Most daily routines involve movement and therefore helping patients to move with minimum breathlessness is an integral part of planning early exercise to promote fitness.

The capacity to communicate needs will be enhanced if the patient is given drinks to maintain a moist mouth, allowing words to be articulated. Liquid food may be the only nourishment that can be taken when breathless and the nurse is in a good position to help (Mackay, 1996a,b). Mouth dryness is a major problem to a breathless patient, made worse by medicines and oxygen therapy. Hydration, attention to oral hygiene and cleaning of nebulizer/inhaler devices are essential if mouth or secondary infections are to be avoided. Fear will influence how a patient copes with the distress of breathlessness and how the nurse demonstrates caring will facilitate the process of communication.

For many patients the acute period is very distressing and difficult decisions arise about the use of respiratory stimulants and/or opiates in the event of deterioration. The nurse can play an important role, spending time with the patient and family, learning what matters to them in respect of a reasonable quality of life. Equally, working with the ward team provides palliative care that increases comfort and minimizes the distress of breathlessness while continuing to instil hope.

In the acute period nursing requires a response to events as they occur, preventing complications whilst optimizing the therapeutic plan; this approach is accompanied by communicating attention to emotional needs, helping a patient feel more reassured and to rehabilitate as recovery begins. The nurses' role in managing the breathless patient and needs is based on continuing to review response to treatment and care. This requires observation and attention to the patient's physical and emotional behaviour including, wherever possible, involving him or her in care and progress; this necessitates a dialogue with other members of the ward team.

Discharging a patient home

Issues

Discharging people from hospital has been recognized as a problem for many years (Armitage, 1985). There is evidence that patient and family needs are not met when patient discharge is unplanned with poor communication between hospital and community staff. There appears to be a number of reasons for this, such as lack of insight into each other's roles and functions; hospital-based care has overshadowed community care and pressure on beds. As far as chronic lung disease is concerned, there has been an emphasis on medical issues, with less understanding about the social aspects of care arising from a patient and family living with chronic illness (Williams, 1993). As lengths of stay in acute care settings diminish and technology for home-based care continues to develop, the scope for expanding nursing at home is considerable (Taylor, 1989). Nurses will need to think more creatively about how the transition from hospital to home can be kept as a continuum for the patient.

Preparing for discharge

PLANNING GOALS

Preparing patients to go home requires attention to be given to needs arising from breathlessness. It is vital to assist the patient to re-establish independence and gain confidence in capacity to move about with the experience of breathlessness. Assessment of how the patient moves around the environment requires practice, through having opportunities to mobilize and undertake a range of activities in hospital, always referring to how this compares with the individual's home situation. For example, how far is it from the sitting room to the lavatory at home? Are the distances in hospital comparable and achievable?

These opportunities provide time to engage the patient in preparing to go home and suggest ideas about when and how to use medicines to ease breathlessness when preparing to move about. This includes how to conserve energy by planning activity and using breathing control. This is where the physiotherapist may advise whilst the patient is in hospital. Initially this exercise may be done using oxygen, which can be delivered by extending the oxygen tube to match the distances to be achieved, thus reducing breathlessness and associated anxiety. Wherever possible, involve the patient in creative strategies to improve the situation rather than thinking about 'problems' – although he or she should be encouraged in problem solving. As discussed by Bury (1991), the term strategy, in contrast to coping, directs attention to the **actions** people take, or what people do in the face of illness, rather than the **attitudes** people develop.

TAKING TREATMENTS

Medicines and use of treatments are important areas in discharge preparation. In patients who are breathless, treatment is time consuming and may have a social impact on everyday routines. Therefore, nursing care is better directed at talking with patients about when they usually take medicines, hearing their opinions about the treatment and enquiring about their ability to collect prescriptions from the chemist. From this it will emerge what difficulties may arise and indeed, whether they plan to take the medicines or have anxieties about the treatment. Employing a personal medicine sheet for several days before leaving hospital in order to practise self-medication gives time to check dexterity and sight. This will give the opportunity to assess comprehension and in some instances recognize illiteracy. For example, hand trembling or small printed labels may lead to difficulties in taking prescribed medicines effectively. Ideally, time should be spent practising how to use a nebulizer at the bedside, fitting masks and nasal cannulae to the face so that both patient and family learn how to use the equipment and can ask additional questions as these arise. During these talking opportunities, the nurse can explore with patients how they would recognize a deterioration in health and what action to take, for example, noticing the colour and consistency of phlegm, recognizing when treatments are not helping and if asthma is present, knowing what the peak flow measurement is when well. Patients may need to be encouraged to contact their general practitioner and also to enter into dialogue about the nature of perceived health changes.

LEARNING ABOUT HEALTH ISSUES

It is worthwhile remembering that, whether discussing medicines, health changes or aspects of rehabilitation with patients and their family, adult learning principles should be kept in mind. Knowles (1973) reminds us that learning is based on four assumptions, which are that people:

- Are self-directed.
- Have accumulated experience.
- Have previous knowledge.
- Are interested in learning through problem solving which is relevant to their life situations.

It is important to remember that, as well as psychosocial factors, the ability to learn may be influenced by physiological factors, for example lethargy or hypercapnia, which may impair understanding and retention of information.

Setting planned time aside to talk in privacy with patients is an opportunity to address their concerns and questions. Questions may arise about health, understanding a diagnosis, prognosis and lifestyle matters. Information is better assimilated if initial concerns are dealt with, followed by relevant educational issues, which should be systematically presented in small chunks, avoiding jargon. Simple diagrams may be helpful to describe emphysema and often there is an interest in explanations on lung anatomy and how the lungs work. The British Lung Foundation has a series of leaflets to supplement verbal information and illustrated children's books, for example the series *How My Body Works* (Barille, 1993), provide stimulating ideas to help express difficult concepts and diagram suggestions that can be incorporated into teaching sessions.

SOCIAL NEEDS

Discharge preparation will include necessary additional services to accommodate social and domestic needs. For example, a person living alone may need shopping, extra personal care or to review financial benefits with a social worker. Another may require adjustments to the home environment to promote mobility, minimizing the experience of breathlessness. This may include a small trolley, facilitating easy access to personal items such as drinks, telephone and hobby material and assisting the patient to move heavier objects from room to room. This is where an occupational therapist may be involved. Here nursing involves a coordination activity and arguably the nurse acts as a broker of services.

In summary, preparing patients to leave hospital is part of the rehabilitation process. Special consideration should be paid to fitness, performing individualized everyday routines and activities, including gaining knowledge and skills with regard to treatments and keeping well. Attending to patients' enquiries will be more meaningful if these are relevant to the reality of life at home.

Discharge

ASSESSMENT

- What capacities does the patient have? What can or can't he or she do?
- What resources does the patient have at home?
- What additional help is needed? (Needs assessment may be necessary, involving a social worker.)
- Which skills or knowledge are required?
- How does the patient feel about going home?

PLAN IMPLEMENTATION

- Set a date for discharge; arrange a ward-based social meeting to discuss the plan.
- Involve the patient and family.
- Provide time to talk about and practise the goals to be achieved.
- Contact other personnel in the community, e.g. Meals on Wheels.

LIAISON

- Confirm verbally and in writing the discharge plan and follow-up care with the general practitioner or community nurse.

ADMINISTRATION

- Arrange transport.
- Arrange follow-up appointments.

- Order medicines.
- Place a copy of the discharge plan on file.

Professional issues

It is reasonable to think that nurses can and should undertake an educational role in rehabilitation. The literature includes many suggestions on what is required to be effective patient teachers, but less is known about how nurses are prepared for this (Close, 1988). New nurse educational curricula place more emphasis on this. Respiratory nurses may be in an ideal position to teach patients because of their interest and specialist knowledge. In this field it is helpful for the patient to have the opportunity to receive information from others in the team, in particular the doctor. A study in Denmark which employed one-to-one teaching sessions from a nurse and doctor set out to improve patients with chronic obstructive pulmonary disease (COPD) with regards to awareness of their illness and feelings of self-control, demonstrating reduced consumption of health services (Tougaard *et al.*, 1992).

Rehabilitation at home

Pulmonary rehabilitation concepts are more readily used by patients and families in their own home and a telephone link is especially valued after discharge. However, continuation of a home programme requires a hospital-based service that is prepared to cooperate with the primary care team.

A starting point therefore is how the respiratory nurse can clarify what pulmonary rehabilitation can provide and what the nurse can offer, continuing the rehabilitation programme within the home. It is useful to employ a framework that clarifies the potential areas of nurse intervention but equally delineates the nurse's function and the potential for overlap or collaboration with other health care workers. It is evident that patients who are living with the physical and psychosocial impact of breathlessness have varied needs which can be analysed within the following conceptual framework of **impairment**, **disability** and **handicap** (World Health Organization, 1980). This framework was employed by Williams and Bury (1989) to analyse the problems of chronic obstructive airways disease and has sharpened our thinking about rehabilitation. Here it is used as a framework to consider nursing intervention.

Since the patient has everyday experiences about feeling intermittently unwell and coping with the unpredictability and uncertainty of this illness, a key intervention is teaching patients how to keep well and solve problems as they arise. Strauss (1975) identified that people and their families have varied social consequences from living with chronic illness and outlined the following significant areas for dealing with chronic illness where nurses can helpfully intervene.

Assistance with carrying out prescribed regimes and managing associated problems

As treatments can be time consuming and restrict peoples lives, offering ideas on how to store and arrange medicines and equipment within easy reach, and how to plan taking them minimizes effort and helps incorporate other social activities into the day, for example suggesting taking a diuretic when returning from shopping.

Following up issues that may have arisen since discharge or as an outcome of taking medicines is discussed further above.

When organizing taking long-term oxygen therapy (LTOT) to cover a 15-h prescription, first acknowledge that this treatment appears restrictive and is a big adjustment. Discuss accrued benefits and emphasize using oxygen during sleep, using time available during meals and nebulizing medicines when taking oxygen via nasal cannulae or whilst sitting reading or watching television. LTOT is often a difficult concept for patients to grasp and anxieties are expressed that they may become dependent. A useful analogy is to compare using oxygen to going out and spending money which it is then necessary to replenish: equally, after being without oxygen for a time, it will be necessary to take oxygen to replace what has been used, emphasizing that it is low dosage. These issues are expanded in a recent article by Heslop and Shannon (1995).

Preventing medical crises and how to manage them when they occur

THE CONTROL OF SYMPTOMS

Patients and their families welcome an opportunity to explore this matter at home; however, talking about a recently experienced medical crisis may be difficult in hospital and during this time it may be more helpful to discuss how to recognize a chest infection and the value of seeking advice promptly. Perhaps a good way to approach managing a medical crisis is to ask what is recalled about recent events leading to admission and what happened when the patient was very breathless. This gives insight into how the situation was managed and previous learning gained, often reassuring the patient and family that they have knowledge that can be used at a future date.

Assistance is needed with practical strategies that alleviate breathlessness using prescribed medicines well (this is why learning effective use of the inhaler is imperative and should be reviewed during hospital admission) and can include ideas about how to use oxygen with a nebulizer, employing breathing control and relaxation strategies. Clearly, if breathlessness can be improved, the patient can think more about what further steps should be taken to control other symptoms, for example a persistent cough, recovery from attempting to expectorate phlegm, dealing with chest pain or other severe symptoms such as osteoporotic pain, insomnia and panic events. Talking through what to do on these occasions and practising breathing control, good positioning and the value of rest can help prepare patients. A home visit is an ideal time to discuss how treatments are being used and when to start reserve antibiotics or oral steroids which will involve liaison with the general practitioner.

Talking through with patients how to manage a variety of scenarios may help them feel more in control of potentially frightening and life-threatening situations. Some may value this written on a card. For some, it may be desirable for a community alarm to be installed so that help is more easily summoned. So often it is the family member who needs support in this area as there is fear about leaving the ill person alone and it is the carer who may become progressively more homebound.

Disability: the consequence of disease limiting the range of activities

The consequence of breathlessness is that patients are unable to do a whole range of practical activities. This causes considerable frustration and distress, which becomes worse as the illness varies on a day-to-day basis, causing uncertainty and making planning difficult. As Fagerhaugh (1975) pointed out in her work with emphysema, patients drew on key mobility resources: **time**, **energy** and **money**. These resources influenced how people organized and developed routines in their day to utilize these resources to best advantage.

Thus, the nurse making a home visit should consider the patient's **environment**, both indoors and outdoors, with respect to getting about.

Key areas to assess and plan for with the patient and family are listed, with restoration of independence in mind so that patients can move about, minimizing breathlessness and potentially keeping fitter.

Indoors

■ Review the immediate environment: height of furniture and its proximity to other essential needs, such as telephone, treatments, nutrition, hobbies and lavatory, assessing how the space can be used to conserve **energy** and **time** while moving about.

■ Assess getting in and out of the bath and rising from the lavatory – are there grab rails nearby?

■ How will food be prepared? Where is it eaten? A small trolley may be helpful.

■ Sleeping area: the patient may need a backrest to sleep upright and help getting in and out of bed. Are an extension telephone and treatments accessible? A bedside urinal can be used to avoid the need to walk to the lavatory.

■ Strategies suggested for moving about: plan moving for washing and dressing, climbing stairs after use of bronchodilators; rest after meals. Discuss the use of oxygen. Talk about clothes which are easier to wear.

■ Review personal care – is help needed with housework? What about personal hygiene and shopping?

■ In conjunction with the above, an exercise plan can be discussed. It should suit the individual (Chapter 4b). These ideas may be explored in hospital and referral to the occupational therapist is helpful.

Outdoors

Most people would prefer to go out and are frustrated about being unable to do things. Exercise plans with realistic goals may help people keep fitter. Establish where a person would choose to go if possible and the distance involved. Issues to consider are:

■ Registering disability.
■ Discuss an exercise plan.
■ Using mobility aids, e.g. a stick.
■ Applying for a taxicard.
■ Wheelchair assessment for longer distances.
■ Assessment for portable oxygen.

It is also useful to check on the need for chiropody and whether other physical, e.g. hernia, or emotional difficulties, e.g. loss of confidence are limiting mobility, which may then be addressed. The nurse may well accompany a patient on initial walks outdoors or involve a family member.

Handicap: resultant social disadvantage

Patients may spend long periods alone or relatives may be limited in going out because of looking after the disabled person. In addition, families living with chronic illness are adjusting to changes, which means confronting emotional, marital and **money** problems – another mobility resource. Issues to consider are:

- Opportunity to talk.
- Funding – what benefits are the family entitled to?
- Potential depression: talk this through and perhaps liaise with the doctor. Some patients need specialized help to cope with panic attacks. Visualization may help.
- Assist with holiday arrangements and moving oxygen concentrators.
- Introduce the patient to the Breathe Easy club.
- Involve a carers' organization to give a spouse a break. A Good Neighbour scheme may help with the practical tasks or provide respite, enabling relatives to have a holiday while the relative is cared for in another setting or has an increase in services.

Carers

Care in the community would not be feasible without the help of informal carers – unpaid assistance given by relatives. The task of caring may be increasingly demanding as impairment worsens. How this care responsibility is perceived and its impact on the carer's social life and family relationships varies. The nature of carer stress and how this can be supported is complex. **Caring** implies both an **activity** and a **relationship**: care comprises a social relationship as well as a physical task (Qureshi, 1986).

Nolan and Grant (1989), drawing on a literature review, summarize what carers perceived they needed from professional services. Areas identified were information, skills training, emotional support and regular respite. Home visiting provides the opportunity to explore these areas and, where possible, assist carers to receive what they need, find solutions to practical problems and have options for themselves too. It is also important that carers receive feedback on caring skills and acknowledgement of their contribution.

> ## The role of the respiratory nurse
>
> To work collaboratively within the wider health care team to provide a service for patients with disabling chest disease, whether in hospital or at home
>
> To provide nursing care that is responsive to health and social needs as a consequence of this illness
>
> To support and educate patients, involving their family, to remain well, using treatments and equipment as well as considering lifestyle adjustments so that they may feel in control of their lives, continuing to live at home
>
> To enable patients with their families to express their emotional needs and what they value as quality of life
>
> To pursue methods to evaluate the effectiveness of nursing practice

Box 9.1

Respite is a difficult area; however, one way around this is offering to teach other institutions, for example showing a nursing home or lay helpers how to use an oxygen concentrator and more often than not giving reassurance and guidance on caring skills. It seems to be valuable to instil confidence and provide a service for institutions outside hospitals so that they are less resistant to offering respite services. Back-up services of this kind need a coordinated response between hospital and community services, funding new approaches to assist families to live better. Carers play a central role in rehabilitation.

Rehabilitation at home is largely subject to assessing sensitively what might provide benefit through a flexible service offering encouragement and reassurance to patients and families. However, it is also complicated by the essential blending of health and social services, which are subject to collaborative work (Heslop and King, 1994).

In conclusion, the nurse has a potentially important contribution to make towards service provision for patients and their families that is responsive to the physical, emotional and social needs of those living with chronic respiratory illness with the associated problems of breathlessness. However, this contribution requires clarification and further evaluation. The development of respiratory nursing as a specialism will for the time being depend on hospital initiatives.

References

Armitage, S. (1985) Hospital to home: discharge referrals, who's responsible? *Nurs. Times* **81**:26–8.

Barille, A. (1993) *How My Body Works: Lungs and Breathing*, vol. 32. Orbis, London.

Baroch, R.M. (1976) *Elements of Rehabilitation in Nursing*. C.V. Mosby, St Louis.

Bury, M.R. (1991) The sociology of chronic illness: a review of research and prospects. *Sociol. Health Illness* **13**:451–68.

Close, A. (1988) Patient education: a literature review. *J. Adv. Nurs.* **13**:203–13.

Cockcroft, A., Heslop, A., Bagnall, P. *et al.* (1987) Controlled trial of a respiratory health worker visiting patients with chronic respiratory disability. *Br. Med. J.* **294**:225–8.

Emerton, A.C. (1986) *Project 2000: A New Preparation for Practice*. UKCC, London.

Fagerhaugh, S. (1975) Getting around with emphysema. In: *Chronic Illness and Quality of Life* (ed A.L. Strauss). C.V. Mosby, St Louis.

Gibbon, B. (1992) The role of the nurse in rehabilitation. *Nurs. Standard* **6**:32–5.

Heslop, A. (1993) Role of the respiratory nurse specialist. *Br. J. Hosp. Med.* **50**:88–9.

Heslop, A., and King, M. (1994) Let's treat body and mind. Collaborative rehabilitation for chronic breathlessness. *Prof. Nurse* **10**:118–92.

Heslop, A., and Shannon, C. (1995) Assisting patients living with long term oxygen therapy. *Br. J. Nurs.* **4**:1123–8.

Knowles, M.S. (1973) *The Adult Learner: A Neglected Species*. Gulf, Houston.

Lertzman, M.M., and Cherniak, R.M. (1976) Rehabilitation of patients with chronic obstructive pulmonary disease. *Am. Rev. Respir. Dis.* **114**:1145–65.

Littlejohn, P., Baveystock, C.M., Parnell, H. *et al.* (1991) Randomised controlled trial of the effectiveness of a respiratory health worker in reducing impairment, disability and handicap due to chronic airflow limitation. *Thorax* **46**:559–64.

Locker, D. (1983) *Disability and Disadvantage. The Consequences of Chronic Illness.* Tavistock, London.

Mackay, L. (1995) The nurse's role in giving nutritional advice. *Prof. Nurse* **10**:427–8.

Mackay, L. (1996a) Nutritional status and chronic obstructive pulmonary disease. *Nurs. Standard* **10**:38–42.

Mackay, L. (1996b) Health education and COPD rehabilitation: a study. *Nur. Standard* **10**:34–9.

Menzies, I.E.P. (1960) *A Case Study in the Functioning of Social Systems as Defence against Anxiety.* Tavistock Institute of Human Relations, London.

Miller A. (1985) Nurse patient dependency – is it iatrogenic? *J. Adv. Nurs.* **10**:63–9.

Ministry of Health and Ministry of Education. (1965) *An Enquiry into Health Visiting on the Field of Work.* HMSO, London.

Myco, F. (1986) A new way of living. *Nurs. Times* **82**:24–7.

Nichols, P.R. (1980) *Rehabilitation Medicine*. Butterworth, London.

Nolan, M.R., and Grant, G. (1989) Addressing the needs of informal carer: a neglected area in nursing practice. *J. Adv. Nurs.* **14**:950–61.

Proctor, S. (1989) The functioning of nursing routines in the management of a transient workforce. *J. Adv. Nurs.* **14**:180–9.

Qureshi, H. (1986) Responses: reciprocity and power relationships. In: *Dependency and Interdependency in Old Age: Theoretical Perspectives and Policy Alternatives* (eds C. Philipson, M. Bernard and R. Strang). Croom Helm, London.

Royal College of Physicians of London. (1981) Disabling chest disease: prevention and cure. *J. R. Coll. Phys. Lond.* **15**:69–87.

Strauss, A.L. (1975) *Chronic Illness and Quality of Life.* C.V. Mosby, St Louis.

Taylor, D. (1989) *Hospital at Home: The Coming Revolution.* King's Fund Centre, London.

Tougaard, L., Krone, T., Sorknaes, A. *et al.* (1992) Economic benefits of teaching patients with chronic obstructive pulmonary disease about their illness. *Lancet* **339**:1517–20.

Waterlow, J. (1985) A risk assessment card. *Nurs. Times* **81**:49–55.

Williams, S.J. (1993) *Chronic Respiratory Illness.* Routledge, London.

Williams, S.J., and Bury M.R. (1989) Impairment, disability and handicap in chronic respiratory illness. *Soc. Sci. Med.* **29**:609–16.

World Health Organization (WHO) (1980) *International Classification of Impairments, Disability and Handicaps.* WHO: Geneva.

Zola, I.K. (1973) Pathways to the doctor: from person to patient. *Soc. Sci. Med.* **7**:677–87.

10. Palliation of non-malignant disease

S. Ahmedzai

Palliative Medicine Section, University of Sheffield, Royal Hallamshire Hospital, Sheffield

Practical Pulmonary Rehabilitation.
Edited by Mike Morgan and Sally Singh.
Published in 1997 by Chapman & Hall, London.
ISBN 0 412 61810 9.

What is palliation?

Palliation is derived from the Latin word *pallium*, which means a short cloak. The related verb *palliare*, to cloak, had the figurative sense of covering up or hiding something, and so in English to palliate came to mean dealing with an issue by hiding it away, rather than removing it or curing the root cause. In medical usage, palliation has acquired the specific meaning of treating a problem associated with a disease (usually a physical symptom, but equally a psychosocial one), without necessarily treating the underlying disease process, and without necessarily affecting the life span.

There are in fact many instances of palliation where the best results are obtained by treating the underlying disease. There are also many types of palliative interventions which can either prolong life, or may run the risk of shortening life span – these are not the primary objectives of treatment but rather are useful or undesirable side-effects, respectively. In some disease processes such as cancer it is relatively easy to separate out curative and palliative interventions. (In practice, many so-called curative therapies in cancer management are really *life prolonging*, as there is no real hope of the patients reverting back to a normal, pre-illness life span.) In non-malignant pulmonary conditions such as chronic obstructive pulmonary disease (COPD), cryptogenic fibrosing alveolitis (CFA) or cystic fibrosis (CF), the situation is somewhat clearer since none of these are strictly curable, and so all treatments – even if they are aggressive, such as lung transplantation, and meant to be life prolonging – are truly palliative, in that they are designed to relieve the subjective distress caused by the disease.

Palliative care and terminal care

In recent years there has been a further medical extension of the word palliative into the field of palliative care. This term has become rather fashionable in the 1990s, and originated as an alternative – in truth, a euphemism – for terminal care. It is not hard to see why another phrase was needed to replace terminal care, since the latter has associations of finality and gloom. It is ironic that the hospice movement itself has played a part in forcing the use of the phrase palliative care, since modern hospices are in reality bright places and have a positive philosophy, in spite of dealing almost exclusively with dying cancer patients.

The World Health Organization (1990) has defined palliative care as:

the active total care of patients whose disease is not responsive to curative treatment. Control of pain, of other symptoms, and of psychological, social and spiritual problems, is paramount. The goal of palliative care is achievement of the best quality of life for patients and their families. Many aspects of palliative care are also applicable earlier in the course of the illness in conjunction with anticancer treatment.

In the UK and Ireland, the concept of palliative care has undergone two further refinements. First, there has been a separation of palliative care services into those which are deemed generic, e.g. those provided by general practitioners, district nurses and some hospitals, and the specialist services, which are the domain of the professional organizations such as hospices, and of Macmillan nurse specialists and hospital-based specialist departments.

The phrase terminal care is used extensively in hospices, but here is meant to refer specifically to the last days or couple of weeks of a patient's life, when there is a discernible change in emphasis of the interventions towards comfort measures (in the past somewhat patronizingly called tender loving care or TLC).

The hospice approach

Mention has already been made of the role of hospices in the provision of palliative care. In the UK these are usually identified as stand-alone establishments – inpatient units (IPUs) which have been purpose built or using modified older buildings. However, as the UK National Council for Hospices and Palliative Care Services (1995) has defined, the hospice approach refers to a philosophy of care rather than a specific building or service and may encompass a programme of care and array of skills deliverable in a wide range of settings. The modern hospice movement has considerable public and professional support for a widespread network of hospices (health service and voluntary) which, increasingly, base their practice on researched knowledge. There is at present no central statutory control of hospice standards in the UK, and it is interesting to note that the National Council adds: 'However, the range and quality of the service are not defined by the use of the term'. In other countries hospice care ranges from religious institutions caring for elderly people to predominantly voluntary home-visiting services.

The relevance of introducing the (British) model of hospice care in this chapter is to highlight its major contribution in the opening up of the previously taboo subject of death and dying. For the past 30 years modern hospices have led the way in using honest communication between patients, family carers and professionals in dealing with issues of accepting an incurable diagnosis, uncertain and terminal prognoses, and facing loss and bereavement. Of course most of this work has been done with advanced cancer, in which the identification of the terminal phase is relatively straightforward, usually linked to metastatic or extensive regional spread.

Many hospices have also opened their doors to patients with progressive neurological diseases such as motor neurone disease and advanced multiple sclerosis. Even in these conditions, it is fairly easy to state when the illness has reached a stage when death is imminent, and patients especially can identify positively with the change in priorities which hospice care facilitates. Indeed, many hospices have waiting lists of such patients who seek admission for respite care (to give their family carers a well-earned rest), for symptom control or for the terminal phase.

Moving beyond cancer

In the past decade hospices have been forced to face other conditions which are as hopeless in terms of prognosis as many malignancies, but which have previously been denied the range and quality of holistic care to which cancer patients have had access. The acquired immunodeficiency syndrome (AIDS) epidemic was thus (somewhat reluctantly at first) seen as a valid call on hospice resources, and indeed there are now several units which are exclusively for human immunodeficiency virus (HIV)/AIDS patients. Some hospices have also started to offer care, in a limited way, to patients with advanced respiratory, cardiac and various degenerative diseases. Usually the trigger for such an admission is the cry for help from a distressed relative or general practitioner who has personal experience of the high level of care given to a cancer patient by a local hospice.

Until now, however, hospice staff (which are often predominantly nurse led) have been diffident about admitting patients suffering from conditions with which they are not familiar. Practical experience, on the other hand, often shows that symptom control and psychosocial aspects of care are very broadly comparable in many end-stage diseases. A large-scale survey of the year before death from cancer and non-cancer causes (evaluated by retrospective interviews with carers) indeed showed that the psychosocial stress of non-malignant diseases may be higher with benign conditions, as they tend to affect older people who have fewer carers to share the burden, and they are also likely to run a more prolonged time-course than many cancers (Seale, 1991). However, there is still considerable grass-roots resistance to the large-scale admission of such groups to hospice care.

At one level this reluctance is understandable and from the point of view of respiratory physicians may even be desirable. It would cause some anxiety among dedicated respiratory teams who have spent considerable time and emotional resources on the rehabilitative care of patients with failing COPD to see them admitted to units where the staff were not knowledgeable about their needs for oxygen, physiotherapy and specific drugs. Injudicious introduction of morphine and other sedative drugs, which are used very extensively in cancer patients attending hospices, could also cause great concern in the minds of respiratory physicians who are less experienced in their use and who are justifiably sceptical of their role. (The use of opioids and sedatives will be discussed in depth later in this chapter.)

There are several reasons therefore why hospice care – whether in an inpatient unit, in home care or at day hospices – has so far had little to offer patients with advanced respiratory diseases. Two major factors may help to change this situation in the coming years. First, the spread of hospital-based palliative care services (often called symptom control or support teams) will make expert palliative care medical and nursing advice readily available to patients who are still attending their respiratory hospital services. Thus, patients admitted to respiratory units for rehabilitation, symptom control or to ease the relatives' burden in advancing disease could be seen by palliative care staff, and be offered advice or possibly be transferred to a specialist palliative care bed. Since these teams tend to have good liaison with community-based services such as local hospices and specialist nurses, on discharge the patient could be more easily introduced to these valuable services. Alternatively, some hospital palliative care teams could see pulmonary rehabilitation patients as outpatients and influence symptom control and the handling of terminal care issues such as discussing prognosis and preparing the family for bereavement from that setting.

The second change is the sociological shift towards a more consumerist attitude which is much in evidence in the UK, in which there is greater demand for patient autonomy and control over the supply of health care resources. This was after all a major factor in the widespread acceptance of hospices for cancer and AIDS patients, and it is not difficult to envisage another surge of interest and ultimately demand for similar high-quality services for other disease categories. Already in the USA there is growing discussion about hospice care needing to cope with the anticipated growth of patients with dementia in our ageing populations. It is interesting to speculate whether, for chronic pulmonary disease patients, there will be integration into mainstream hospices alongside cancer and neurological disease sufferers. Respiratory physicians, nurses and paramedical staff involved in pulmonary rehabilitation programmes have an important part to play in influencing this trend. There should be open channels between the two types of service for clinical communication, education, joint research and audit to identify ways of improving care for patients and families irrespective of their location.

Where can palliative care help?

In the management of malignant disease the concept of palliation and increasingly of palliative care is well established. But in the field of pulmonary medicine these are not often specifically brought to bear in the care of patients with advancing benign disease. This is partly because, as described above, palliative and hospice services have long sought to restrict themselves to cancer patients to the virtual exclusion of other diseases, but also because clinicians working with lung disease are not familiar with the benefits of the palliative care approach.

What could be the benefits? And which patients could gain? It is perhaps too easy to reply that all patients with lung disease could benefit from palliative interventions. Although that might be true in the literal sense, and indeed I have argued above that much of the management of chronic lung disease is palliative since the underlying disease cannot be eradicated and the patient's life span is not restored to normal, it is clearly neither feasible nor desirable for pulmonary services to change all their practices to a hospice-type approach. It is important for the morale of many patients to feel that they are being cared for in an environment where active – even aggressive – treatments are being pursued, possibly in the context of research programmes, so that hope for an improved quality of life and a longer life is maintained.

Symptom control and total pain

Improvement in symptom control is clearly the main benefit of a palliative approach. It is necessary to take a broad view, however, when considering which symptoms the patient may be suffering from, and to what extent they trouble the patients and the family. In cancer palliative care, it has long been recognized that, although pain is often seen as the major fear of patients, it is not only the physical sensation of pain which causes distress. The concept of total pain is a brilliantly simple but far-reaching idea that has been one of the major contributions of Dame Cicely Saunders (1967), one of the founders of the modern hospice movement. In this concept, chronic cancer pain is deconstructed to at least five separate and interactively linked components: the physical, psychological, social, spiritual (existential) and financial elements. At a particular time, the patient's experience may be dominated by any one of these aspects, or several could be working and even aggravating each other.

Furthermore,the balance of factors can change during the illness; for example, in the early stages the physical expression of nociception can predominate, but later on, psychological consequences such as anxiety and depression can be added, and in the more advanced stages the patient may be overcome by existential questions such as 'Why me?' and 'What is the purpose of this suffering?' Although not originally caused by the pain, these questions, if unanswered or unshared, can compound it. All through a chronic illness such as cancer, the social impact of pain is evident in the restrictions it places on mobility, occupation, maintenance of role and social or sexual relationships.

The purpose of introducing the cancer total pain concept here is that it can be easily transferred to chronic pulmonary disease and to other symptoms, such as dyspnoea. Palliation of the physical distress will be discussed later: the reader is asked now to consider the other impacts of chronic symptoms on respiratory disease patients and their carers. It may be that with severe end-stage disease, there are very few opportunities for further symptom improvement or gain in mobility. At this stage it is not uncommon for patients to be told – either bluntly or with regret – that nothing more can be done. Trevor Clay (1994), a senior nurse manager who also suffered from chronic and terminal lung disease, wrote:

> One of my preoccupations is the language we all use and one of my ambitions is to dissuade health professionals from saying 'there's nothing more that can be done'. Apart from the devastating effect it has on people, it is simply not true. What is meant is that there is no cure, no magic, but there is always something that can be done. This isn't just political correctness, but goes to the core of what we need to be addressing.

The clinician who is caring for a patient with advancing pulmonary disease therefore has to be aware of the other kinds of suffering that may be going on in the patient's life, and how they may be impacting on the family and circle of friends. Even if life cannot be prolonged, or symptoms reduced any further without excessive side-effects, the psychological, social and existential concerns of the patient may still be quite amenable to palliation. As Shee (1995) has written, 'Respiratory medicine can learn from palliative medicine in considering the meaning of dyspnoea in the context of life-threatening illness. It can be extremely therapeutic for patients, often for the first time, to express their feelings and fears (e.g. fear of dying). One hears phrases such as "nobody understands".'

Multidisciplinary teamwork

Of course the respiratory worker – whether doctor, nurse, physiotherapist or other professional – does not have to possess all the skills to attend to all of these concerns. In the hospice approach of modern palliative care services, it is acknowledged that the secret to its success is the application of well-managed interdisciplinary teamwork. The multiprofessional team which can be brought to bear on the patient and family can be large, but again not all members need to be full-time or even professionally attached to the pulmonary service. It is sufficient to know that serious psychological problems, which a nurse or physiotherapist may be able to detect more easily than a doctor, could be referred on to a sympathetic psychologist or professional counselling service, such as some hospices run. Social workers are less integrated into hospital clinics now than they used to be, and it may be easier to arrange access via the community teams.

Support of families

Another parallel with the world of palliative care is the emphasis given there on the burden of illness which also falls on the carers, especially on elderly wives or husbands, or working children who may have to take time off to provide care for an increasingly dependent parent. Thus, the clinical team treating a patient with progressive pulmonary disability would be failing in their holistic role if they ignored the family's and friends' stress and morbidity. In exploring the stresses on informal carers, the respiratory care team may unearth major conflicts within what is externally seen as a supportive family. Patients who are reluctant to give up previously important roles, such as earning a significant income or house-keeping, may cause particularly difficult problems for other members of the family who have to take these roles over without thanks. It is also easy to assume that couples or elderly parents and adult chidren are committed to each other: there may have been a long-standing family division and it is not reasonable to expect others automatically to adopt a loving, caring attitude towards a debilitated, increasingly dependent and possibly cantankerous relative. Once again, these problems cannot be resolved by respiratory clinicians, but they should try to identify their existence and then refer them back to the general practitioner or to social workers. If the pulmonary programme has the benefit of specialist respiratory nurses, then they could be very helpful in this role, much as Macmillan nurse specialists are in the continuing care of cancer patients in the community.

Existential and spiritual distress

The existential or spiritual concerns which patients with end-stage disease may reveal can be very challenging for clinicians. Even if they do not consider it 'their job' to help the patient with them, it is still helpful for professionals to allow patients sufficient time and privacy to confide these issues. In hospices too, few professionals consider themselves skilled to deal with spiritual problems, but they are trained to listen sympathetically in such a way that the patient feels tremendous relief at sharing the burden of worries. Spiritual concerns themselves are usually not religious in the sense of focusing on doubts about God, or life after death, etc. In modern western society the more frequent doubts are about 'Why me?' and 'What did I do to deserve this?' Guilt about smoking or other forms of self-abuse and anger over previous working conditions can also disturb the patient's equilibrium. There are, naturally, no easy answers for these questions – that is not the point, because few patients would accept formulaic answers from professionals anyway. Rather, it is the knowledge that the professional seems to care, and tries to find time to allow the expression of such feelings, that brings satisfaction to the patient.

Where the questions do focus on religious matters, it is of course essential to make available the appropriate minister, priest or other professional. It is easy to assume that a Catholic, Jew or Muslim living in a pluralistic society such as modern urban Britain is in touch with his or her religious leader – indeed, the very cause of spiritual distress may be the need to reconcile oneself, before death, with a long abandoned religion.

Planning terminal care

For most patients with a progressive pulmonary disease, there will be a time when it is clear that all attempts to prolong life are fruitless, and that the prognosis is now very limited. Often this occurs after an acute event, such as an infective exacerbation or a severe episode of cardiac decompensation. These situations may be easier to recognize and respond to, because the sudden deterioration is apparent to all, including the patient, the family and the professional team. Even so, there may be some reluctance, usually on the part of one or other family member, or a professional who feels that active treatment should always be pursued, to accept that the end is near, and that the clinical approach should turn to one aimed at comfort. It is important to recognize when one of the key players (who might, of course, be the patient) is blocking the inevitable transition towards terminal care, and to try and understand the motives for this.

Acceptance of terminal stage

The patient may, understandably, be resistant to the idea that he or she has finally reached the 'end of the line'. Usually this arises when during the weeks and months prior to this pathophysiological change in status, the patient has been denied the opportunity to explore the possibility of dying from the lung disease, and coming to terms with that. This implies addressing the psychological and existential concerns referred to above. In pulmonary services where suitably trained staff are not made available to open up and guide the patient through such deep waters of self-discovery, then the acceptance of the terminal prognosis will be more problematic for some individuals. This is not to declare that all patients should accept the fact of their death. The reaction to being faced with a fatal prognosis and the stages of preparation for death, which have been described sociologically and psychologically by Kübler-Ross and others, include numbness, anger, denial, fighting spirit and, for some, acceptance. People can find themselves at more than one stage at the same time and it may quite appropriate for some individuals to spend their last days and hours in flat denial and fighting against death, as they had always fought against unpleasant situations in earlier life. Such a death may be uplifting for professionals to observe, providing that the patient's feelings do not cause severe distress to the relatives.

Another, perhaps more common scenario is where the patient has quietly or overtly acquiesced and is awaiting death. He or she may even openly talk about it with the doctors and nurses, perhaps asking for treatments to be withdrawn and – a situation that many clinicians dread – ask for measures to be taken to speed up the process. It is beyond the scope of this chapter to discuss the issues surrounding euthanasia and assisted suicide. It is important for all professionals dealing with incurable and fatal diseases to be aware of the growing literature on this subject, and especially on the topic of advanced directives (Age Concern Working Party, 1988). Although these are not legally binding at present in the UK, it is nevertheless very helpful for patients some time before they enter the terminal stage to have written down how they would like to be treated – aggressively to maintain life at all costs, with minimal interference from drips and machinery to preserve personal ideas of dignity, or somewhere in between. Even if a patient has made an advance directive, and no doubt increasingly older people are being advised to in our society, the professional team should always consider the possibility that patients may change their mind at the last minute.

Family conflicts

Quite often the patient and professional carers are agreed on the appropriate path to be followed in far-advanced disease, but the family carers are at odds with this course. Sometimes it is one member, perhaps a wife or husband; or a dutiful daughter who has given up years to look after a dependent parent; or in the case of younger patients with end-stage conditions such as cystic fibrosis, the parents. Less frequently, the pulmonary care team is faced with a family which is more or less equally divided on the issue of terminal care versus more life-prolonging therapy: often this situation reflects long-standing divisions in families, and may even have brought together a family which had for decades been widely scattered and out of communication with each other. A particularly difficult scenario for British doctors to deal with is when a family member appears from a country like the USA, demanding to know what further measures are being taken and threatening legal action if they see the care being withdrawn or less active compared to what they would have experienced 'back home'. All these situations require very careful handling, so as not to upset the patient as well as to avoid formal complaints or litigation. A social worker should be involved, and the family members' own personal motives should be sought on why they are insisting on prolonging active treatment (or the opposite if they are demanding withdrawal of therapy against the advice of the professionals). Often the motivation is altruistic, such as the relative's desire to do the best for the patient, based on discussions and memories of what he or she had wished for in previous life; other times relatives are expressing their own anxieties about confronting death.

Role of the primary care team

In the situations described above, it is likely that the patient is in hospital for the management of an acute episode. It is quite easy, therefore, for the pulmonary care team to ignore the important role of the general practitioner and district nurses in the decision-making process, and even the practical care of the patient. In modern urban communities it may no longer be the case that the general practitioner is familiar with all his or her chronically ill patients and is seen by them as the main carer and confidant. Even so, the general practitioner has a vital role in maintaining the mental and physical health of not only the patient but also other family members who may be on the general practitioner's list. Thus, the primary care team should be consulted and even invited to participate in case conferences in which the immediate and longer-term care is being planned for a terminally ill pulmonary patient.

Choosing the place of death

One issue in which the general practitioner has a major role to play is the choice of place for the patient's eventual death. Even if the patient has formed an opinion on this (and there are many who still do not, either because of lack of preparation or an inner reluctance to face the issue), there are many factors which may conspire to modify this choice. Many people, when well and enjoying a stable life with their family, will state that they wish to die at home. In severe illness, however, and when the relatives have borne a great burden of caring and perhaps even financial hardship, patients may change their mind; or else, circumstances force a move to hospital, against their expressed wishes. It is vital for the pulmonary care team to try and ascertain what the patient's and the family's views are on the place of death, and to review this at intervals as the disease progresses into the terminal phase. Consultation with the general practitioner and district nurse will be very helpful in determining if the choice is realistic, and will also enable special provisions to be made in the case of a home death. It is likely that the patient will already have a variety of aids by this stage, such as commode, walking frame or wheelchair, perhaps a hospital-type bed, as well as oxygen. Sometimes, because of housing circumstances, it is just not possible to bring all the necessary equipment into the house, or the accommodation will not allow for the patient's bed to be moved to a suitable room.

Bereavement support

The primary care team also plays a major role in the bereavement support of surviving relatives; the hospital team can also identify family members who appear to be having exceptional difficulties in adjustment during the terminal phase, and to bring their anticipatory grieving needs to the attention of the general practitioner, social worker or bereavement counselling service. Some hospices may offer grief support to patients' families, even if the patient is not referred to the service. Cruse is a UK charitable organization which can be very helpful in helping people adjust to bereavement. It is important for both hospital staff and the primary care team to be able to recognize when a family carer is having exceptional difficulty in preparing for bereavement, and appropriate referral should be made to a psychiatry or psychology service if there is thought to be a risk of pathological grief, when the possibility of self-neglect or even suicide is raised.

Crisis management at the end of life

Even though many patients may choose to die at home, it is inevitable that medical crises may occur in the terminal stages, for which the appropriate response is urgent readmission to hospital. If the primary care team is well prepared, trained and equipped, it may be possible to manage some acute crises at home. However, most occurrences of acute respiratory failure or cardiac failure, such as those due to infection, lead to admission, often at night or at weekends when the patient's usual general practitioner is unavailable. The hospital team should be familiar with the patient and should, above all, be informed about whether the patient should be treated actively and possibly even resuscitated in the event of acute arrest. Bearing in mind what was noted above about the likely increase in living wills and advance directives, patients themselves or their relatives may draw to the medical team's attention a prior decision *not* to be resuscitated.

The medical management of distressing symptoms in acute crises is detailed in Boxes 10.1–10.8. There is a growing acceptance of drugs such as morphine in the terminal phase of chronic respiratory disease, overcoming the blind objection of the past which was based on physiological rather than on palliative (or humanitarian) grounds.

Palliation of specific symptoms

There are many textbooks and manuals of symptom control for the palliative care of patients with malignancy. It is doubtful whether these are consulted very frequently by clinicians in other fields of health care; this leads to the sad inevitability of unnecessarily unrecognized and unrelieved distress in non-cancer patients. It is not feasible to translate here all the accumulated knowledge from cancer-based symptom control to the pulmonary field, and Boxes 10.1–10.8 consist of brief extracts of this knowledge base wherever there are relatively easy gains to be made in the improvement of the pulmonary patient's quality of life. The reader should be aware, however, that the scientific basis of these recommendations is very thin, because the research evidence, and even the empirical clinical practice, is greatly lacking.

The guidelines given in Boxes 10.1–10.8 for symptom control are based on the further reading list, especially the chapter on respiratory problems in the (rather weighty) *Oxford Textbook of Palliative Medicine* and Regnard and Tempest's excellent little notebook on symptom control. For explanation and detailed references to the recommendations in the

267

boxes, the reader is advised to consult these volumes, or, better, to contact the local specialist palliative medicine service (hospice or hospital support team).

Causes of dyspnoea in advanced and terminal disease

Pulmonary
Obstructive airways disease
Fibrotic lung disease
Malignancy
Infection
Pneumothorax
Pulmonary embolism
Pleural effusion
Cardiac
Heart failure
Pericardial effusion
Neuromuscular
Motor neurone disease
Diaphragmatic failure
Chest-wall muscle weakness
Haematological
Anaemia
Polycythaemia
Psychological
Hyperventilation

Box 10.1

Overall management strategies for dyspnoea

Drug therapy
Ventilatory support
Oxygen therapy
Physiotherapy
Nursing care
Psychological support

Box 10.2

Drug therapy of dyspnoea

Airways obstruction
Bronchodilators
Methylxanthines
Corticosteroids
Respiratory stimulants

Infection
Antibiotics
Mucolytics

Cardiac
Diuretics
Angiotensin-converting enzyme
    inhibitors
Digoxin

Malignancy
Cytotoxics
Hormones

Non-specific
Opioids
Benzodiazepines
Buspirone
Antidepressants
Cannabinoids

Box 10.3

Using morphine in advanced respiratory disease

Actions
Anxiolytic
Improves exercise tolerance
Reduces sensation of dyspnoea
Hypnotic
N.B.: Rarely produces euphoria in medical usage

Side-effects
Sedation
Cognitive impairment (very variable – intolerable in some; others may drive and have no discernible problem)
Constipation (can be severe and unremitting)
Nausea (usually lasts a few days only)

Other risks
Respiratory depression (not usually a problem if dose is built up *slowly*)
Psychological dependence (addiction – usually not a problem in medical usage)
Physical dependence (may produce withdrawal syndrome if drug is stopped abruptly)

Recommended use of morphine
Test dose of 5 mg instant-release morphine
Titrate up dose using 4-hourly instant-release form
Convert to slow-release form (12- or 24-hourly) only when titration is stable
Many patients would prefer to take slow-release morphine by night and 1–2 doses of instant-release form p.r.n. by day

269

Box 10.4

Management of cough

Bronchodilators

Nebulized saline

Mucolytic

Opioids
    Codeine
    Morphine or methadone

Nebulized local anaesthetic
    For severe unproductive cough, try 5 ml of 2% lignocaine at
    night or b.i.d.
    Beware of bronchospasm in asthmatics
    Risk of aspiration unlikely after 1 h

Physiotherapy

Nursing position

N.B.: Try stopping angiotensin-converting enzyme inhibitors!

Box 10.5

Overall management strategies for pain

Mild pain
Paracetamol

Moderate pain
Weak opioid, e.g. codeine, dihydrocodeine, tramadol

Severe pain
Strong opioid, e.g. morphine, transdermal fentanyl

Localized pain, e.g. rib fracture
Nerve block
Transcutaneous electrical nerve stimulation (TENS)

Chronic pain and depression
Antidepressant

Box 10.6

Other troublesome symptoms in chronic lung disease

Anorexia/cachexia
High-energy/protein foods and supplements
Appetite stimulants:
   Progestogens, e.g. megestrol
   Corticosteroids (but note short action and fluid retention)
Weakness
Treat anaemia
Improve anorexia
Physiotherapy
Occupational therapy
Aids for daily living
Constipation (especially if on opioid)
High-fibre food and bulking agents
Stimulant and lubricant laxatives
Regular nursing checks for impaction
Poor sleep
Treat nocturnal cough
Anxiolytic
Hypnotic
Opioid

Box 10.7

Psychological distress

Anxiety
Benzodiazepine
Buspirone
Low-dose morphine
Counselling
Depression
Antidepressants
Treat unresolved pain
Consider 'spiritual pain'
Counselling

Box 10.8

References

Age Concern Working Party. (1988) *The Living Will*. Edward Arnold, London.

Clay, T. (1994) How to keep the customer satisfied. *Thorax* **49**:279–80.

National Council for Hospice and Specialist Palliative Care Services. (1995) *Specialist Palliative Care: A Statement of Definitions*. Occasional paper 8. National Council for Hospice and Specialist Palliative Care Services, London.

Saunders, C. (1967) *The Management of Terminal Illness*. Edward Arnold, London.

Seale, C. (1991) Death from cancer and death from other causes: the relevance of the hospice approach. *Palliative Med.* **5**:12–19.

Shee, C.D. (1995) Palliation in chronic respiratory disease. *Palliative Med.* **9**:3–12.

World Health Organization. (1990) *Cancer Pain Relief and Palliative Care*. World Health Organization, Geneva.

Further reading

Ahmedzai, S. (1988) Respiratory distress in the terminally ill patient. *Respir. Dis. Practice* **5**:20–9.

Ahmedzai, S. (1993) Palliation of respiratory symptoms. In: *Oxford Textbook of Palliative Medicine* (eds D. Doyle, G. Hanks, N. MacDonald). Oxford Medical Publications, Oxford, pp. 349–78.

Light, R.W., Muro, J.R., Sato, R.I. *et al.* (1959) Effects of oral morphine on breathlessness and exercise tolerance in patients with chronic obstructive pulmonary disease. *Am. Rev. Respir. Dis.* **139**:126–33.

Petty, T.L. (1987) Dealing with final stages of disease. In: *Chronic Obstructive Pulmonary Disease: Current Concepts* (eds J.E. Hodgkin and T.L. Petty). WB Saunders, Philadelphia, pp. 279–93.

Regnard, C., and Ahmedzai, S. (1991) Dyspnoea in advanced nonmalignant disease – a flow diagram. *Palliative Med.* **5**:56–60.

Regnard, C.F.B., and Tempest, S. (1992) *A Guide to Symptom Relief in Advanced Cancer*. Haigh & Hochland, Manchester.

Tywcross, R. (1995) *Introducing Palliative Care*. Radcliffe Medical Press, Oxford.

Appendix A
Abbreviations

ACBT	active cycle of breathing techniques
AIDS	acquired immunodeficiency syndrome
AT	anaerobic threshold
ATP	adenosine triphosphate
BMI	body mass index
BPQ	Breathing Problems Questionnaire
CF	cystic fibrosis
CFA	cryptogenic fibrosing alveolitis
COPD	chronic obstructive pulmonary disease
CRDQ	Chronic Respiratory Disease Questionnaire
CT	computed tomographic
DIT	diet-induced thermogenesis
FET	forced expiration technique
FEV_1	forced expiratory volume in 1 s
Fio_2	fractional concentration of inspired oxygen
FLS	forward lean sitting
FRC	functional residual capacity
FVC	forced vital capacity
GER	general exercise reconditioning
HIV	human immunodeficiency virus
IBW	ideal body weight
IMT	inspiratory muscle training
IPPV	intermittent positive-pressure ventilation
IPU	inpatient unit
LTOT	long-term oxygen therapy
MAC	mid-arm circumference
MAMC	mid-arm muscle circumference
MBC	maximal breathing capacity
MRC	Medical Research Council
MSVC	maximum sustained ventilatory capacity
MVV	maximal voluntary ventilation
NHP	Nottingham Health Profile
NIPPV	nasal intermittent positive-pressure ventilation

Paco$_2$	partial pressure of arterial carbon dioxide
Pao$_2$	partial pressure of arterial oxygen
Pdi	transdiaphragmatic pressure
QOL	quality of life
REE	resting energy expenditure
RV	residual volume
Sao$_2$	oxygen saturation
SF-36	Short Form-36
SGRQ	St George's Respiratory Questionnaire
SIP	Sickness Impact Profile; sustainable inspiratory pressure
SIT	stress inoculation training
T_i	inspiratory time
TLC	total lung capacity; tender loving care
TLCO	transfer factor for lung carbon monoxide
TSF	triceps skinfold
T_{tot}	length of breathing cycle
VAS	visual analogue score
V_E	ventilation
$V_{E_{max}}$	maximal ventilation
Vo$_2$	oxygen consumption
Vo$_{2max}$	maximal oxygen consumption
Vo$_{2peak}$	peak oxygen consumption

Appendix B
Useful addresses

Air Transport Users Committee
2nd Floor
Kingsway House
103 Kingsway
London
WC2B 6QX
(0171) 242 3382

ASH (Action on Smoking and Health)
5/11 Mortimer Street
London
W1N 7RH

Breathe Easy
c/o British Lung Foundation (see below)

British Lung Foundation
78 Hatton Garden
London
ECIN 8JR
(0171) 831 5831

British Red Cross
National Headquarters
9 Grosvenor Crescent
London
SW1X 7EJ
(0171) 235 5454

DIAL UK
The National Association of Disablement
   Information and Advice Lines
(01302) 310123

Park Lodge
St Catherine's Hospital
Tickhill Rd
Doncaster
DN4 8QN

Handihols
12 Ormonde Avenue
Rochford
Essex
SS4 1QW
(01702) 548257

Holiday Department
Disabled Living Services
Redbank House
4 St Chad's St
Cheetham
Manchester
M8 8QA
(0161) 832 3678

QUIT
The National Society of Non-Smokers
Latimer House
40–48 Hanson St
London
W1P 7DE

RADAR
Royal Association for Disability and
   Rehabilitation
25 Mortimer St
London
W1N 8AB
(0171) 637 5400

Index

Note: page numbers in *italics* refer to tables, those in **bold** refer to figures.

Acetazolamide 226
Active cycle of breathing techniques (ACBT) 167–8
Activity avoidance 201
Acupuncture 175
  smoking cessation 221
Adenosine triphosphate resynthesis 69, 71, 72
Advanced directives 264, 267
Aerobic training 14, 82
  components 92
  cycling 86
  duration of session 91–2
  effective regimen 90
  effectiveness measurement 95–6
  exercise prescription 87, **88**, 89–90
  frequency 92, **93**
  heart rate 89–90
  intensity 85–6, 89, 90–1
  lactate concentration measurement 87
  maintenance exercises 94
  patient categorizing 91
  progression 93–4
  regimens 86
  response 84–6
  supplemental oxygen 94, **95**
  symptom-limited 89
  $V_{O_{2peak}}$ measurement 87
  V_{O_2} indirect measures 87
  walking 86
AIDS, hospice care 258
Air travel, respiratory disease 231–2
Airflow generation 84
Airflow limitation and
  arm activity 119
  oxidative enzymes 118
  peripheral muscle strength 118
  rehabilitation programmes 215
  weight-lifting training 122–3
Airflow obstruction, chronic 218
Airway
  function in COPD 5
  hyperreactive 158
  resistance in COPD 108
Alarm systems 210
Albumin 138
  visceral protein status 144

Alveolar gas exchange 70
American College of Chest Physicians Committee on Pulmonary Rehabilitation 8
American Thoracic Society 8, 21
Aminophylline 226
Anaerobic threshold in COPD 86
Anger 263
Ankle oedema 218
Antibiotics 226
Anticholinergic drugs 222, 223
Anxiety 158, 271
  attitude changing 172, 173, 174
  management 187, 195–7
Appetite, poor 151–2
Arm
  activity 119
  fat area (AFA) 142–3
  muscle area (AMA) 142–3
Arm training 75, 77
  supported/unsupported 121
  see also Upper-extremity training
Asthma
  anticholinergics 222, 223
  β-agonist drugs 222, 223
  bronchodilators 221
  clinical guidelines 3
  corticosteroids 225
  emotional problems 58
  exercise training 74
  inspiratory muscle training 110
  onset 3
  peak flow measurement 216
  physical problems 58
  quality of life 58
  rehabilitation programmes 215
  smoking history 218
Attitude of mind, time management 198
Autogenic drainage 168–9
Avoidance strategy 196
Awareness of thought processes 197

β-agonist drugs 222, 223
Barriers, physical/social 184
Barthel Index *188*

Behaviour
  modification 174
  patterns 181
Behavioural strategy in anxiety management 195–7
Benefit system 209
Bereavement 258
  support 266
Bioelectrical impedance 138, 143–4
Body composition
  assessment 138–9
  fat mass 137, 138
  fat-free mass 137, 138
  monitoring 149–50
  normal 138
  nutritional assessment 137–9
  reserves 138
Body mass index (BMI) 134–5, *136*
Body weight
  nutritional assessment 134–5, *136*
  see also Obesity; Weight loss
Bone density assessment 138
Borg scale 30
  symptom-limited exercise training 89
Breathe Easy groups *see* Self-help group; Support groups
Breathing
  active cycle of breathing techniques (ACBT) 167–8
  components 84
  cycle duration (Ttot) 102
  deep 167
  diaphragmatic 164
  patterns in breathlessness 218
  pursed-lip 165, 218
  retraining 164
  work 157–62, **163**, 164–5
Breathing control 162, 164–5
  active cycle of breathing techniques (ACBT) 167
  activity 165
  learning 164
  strategies 248
Breathing Problems Questionnaire 38, 50, *52*, 54, **55**, 56, 60
  subscales 56–7, 59
Breathlessness 6
  alleviation strategies 248
  assessment 28–31
  breathing patterns 218
  chronic airflow limitation 118
  conceptual framework 246
  energy conservation 201
  forward lean sitting position 159
  goal planning 243
  perception 84, 89
  physiotherapy 156, 157–62, **163**, 164–5
  respiratory nursing 240–2
  see also Dyspnoea
Bronchiectasis
  antibiotics 226

rehabilitation programme 21
  secretion clearance 169
Bronchoconstriction 158
Bronchodilators 221–2
  nebulized 224
  prescription 9
Buildings
  adaptations 188
  architectural adaptations 210
  design 184

Calorie intake 147–8
  target 148
Canadian Occupational Performance Measure *188*
Carbon dioxide arterial partial pressure ($Paco_2$) 27, 162, 227, 229
  breathing control 165
Carbon dioxide production (Vco_2) 36
  arm activity 119
Cardiac function in COPD 70
Cardiac output
  activity 69–70
  maximal 69
Carers 250–1
  organizations 250
Chest
  clapping 169–70
  compression with shaking and/or vibration 170
  hyperinflation reduction 160
  percussion 169
  radiography 146, 216
  trauma 21
Chronic obstructive pulmonary disease (COPD) 2
  aerobic training 90–1
  airway function 5, 221–6
  anaerobic threshold 86
  ankle oedema 218
  antibiotics 226
  anticholinergics *222*, 223
  arm training 75, 77
  β-agonist drugs 223
  breathing pattern 158
  breathlessness 28
  bronchodilators 221–2, 224
  cigarette smoking 218
  clinical features 217–18
  corticosteroids 224–6
  development 3
  endurance 72
    training 73–6, 109
  energy balance in malnourished patients 130–1
  exercise
    aerobic 90–1
    incremental test 83
    intensity 78
    limitations 83–4, *85*
    rehabilitation 66

symptom-limited training 89
  therapeutic 76–8
  tolerance 83
food intake 131
functional capacity decline 68, 82
gas exchange 26–7
hyperinflation 108
ideal body weight (IBW) 134
impairment 4–5
inactivity 68
inspiratory muscle training 108–9
lung function measurement 216–17
malabsorption 131–2
malnutrition 128–34
  energy balance 130–1
  reversal 133–4
management 3, 10
medical treatment 221–6
natural history 217–18
nutrition 128, 134
occupational therapy 180, 181
overweight patient 147–8
oxygen
  limitation 35
  uptake capacity 70
palliation 256
patient motivation 39
performance 182–5
  skills 182–3
polycythaemia 218
referral 21
rehabilitation programme 215
  compliance 39–42
resting energy expenditure (REE) 132–3
role effects 182–3
sexual activity 205
theophyllines *222*, 223
treatment 218–19
vicious circle **82**
volition 183–4
weight loss 129, 218
Chronic Respiratory Disease Questionnaire 38, 50,
    52–3, 56, 60, *188*
  subscales 56–7
  upper-extremity training 122
Chronically Sick and Disabled Persons Act (1970) 210
Cigarette smoking *see* Smoking
Cognitive therapy 195, 197
Cognitive-motivational factors in patient compliance
    40
Communication 188, 208–10
  hospice care 257
  hospital and community staff 242
  needs 242
  respiratory medicine 239–40
  respiratory nurse 242
Community staff 242

Compliance
  cognitive-motivational factors 40
  goals 41
  improvement 40–1
  information provision 41
  rehabilitation programme 39–42
  self-reporting 42
  somatic factors 40
  tailoring 41
Compressors, physiotherapist education role 172
Computed tomography (CT) 216
Confidence 66
  physiotherapist role 173–4
Cor pulmonale 143, 232
Corticosteroids
  inhaled 225–6
  oral 221, 224–5
Coughing 218
  management 270
  suppression 166
Creatinine height index 139
Crisis management 267
Cryptogenic fibrosing alveolitis, palliation 256
Cultural prejudice 184–5
Cycle
  endurance in upper-extremity training 122
  ergometer test 32, **34**, 36
Cycling 96
Cystic fibrosis
  active cycle of breathing techniques (ACBT) 167
  gastrostomy 150
  inspiratory muscle training 110
  palliation 256
  respiratory muscle endurance 108
  secretion clearance 171

Daily living tasks 184–5
Death, choosing place 266
Deconditioning
  avoidance 66–8
  COPD 82
Dementia 259
Depression 250
Desensitization, systematic 196
Diabetes mellitus, pulmonary rehabilitation 128
Diaphragm
  configuration 28–9
  contractile properties during hyperinflation 108
  contraction force 159
  length-tension relationship 159
  positioning 159
  strength 101
Diet in endurance training 70–1
Dietary counselling 149
Dietary history 145, 146
Dietitian 43, 149
  rehabilitation programme 144

Disability 7
  assessment 12
  conceptual framework of breathlessness 246
  definition 4, 5
  estimates 9
  fitness 249
  getting out from home 249–50
  inability to do range of activities 248–50
  onset **6**
  reduction 14
  residual 10
Discharge from hospital 242–6
  administration 245–6
  assessment 245
  goal planning 243
  health issues 244
  liaison 245
  medicines 243–4
  plan implementation 245
  preparation 243–5
  recognition of deterioration 244
  social needs 245
  treatments 243–4
Disease education 214–15
  airway function improvement 221–6
  chronic airflow limitation 215–16
  COPD
    clinical features/natural history 217–18
    medical treatment 221–6
    treatment 218–19
  lung structure/function 216–17
  smoking cessation 219–21
Distraction in anxiety management 196
Distress 271
  patient 263
Diversion in anxiety management 196
Doxapram 226
Dual-energy X-ray absorptiometry 138
Dyspnoea 28, 29–30
  awareness 84
  causes 268
  COPD 182, 218
  drug therapy 269
  exercise 14–15
  fear 157
  inspiratory muscle training 109
  management strategies 268
  measurement 53
  ratings 30–1
  relief 161
  scales 29–30
  symptom intensity 30
  see also Breathlessness

Education
  anxiety management 195
  energy conservation 201
  health issues 244
  lifestyle management 187
  physiotherapy 171–4
  time management 198–9
Effort magnitude 30
Emotional problems 250
Emphysema
  breathing control 165
  diaphragm weight 130
  head-down position 162
  surgery 234–5
Endurance test 36–7
  submaximal 96
Endurance training 66
  adapatation 76
  arm training 121
  capacity 69
  COPD 73–6
  diet 70–1
  evaluation 71–2
  exercise 92
  intensity 90–1
  limitations 70–2
  muscle changes 72
  normal individuals 72
  physiological stress 72
  studies 73–4
  $V_{O_{2max}}$ 72
Energy balance 66
Energy balance
  negative energy expenditure 132–3
  malabsorption 131–2
  malnutrition in COPD 130–1
Energy conservation 187
  education 201
  home 249
  physiotherapist education role 172
Energy expenditure, negative energy balance 132–3
Enteral feeding, supplementary 150
Environment 184–5
  adaptation 203–4
  energy conservation 201, 203–4
  home 248
Equipment provision
  accessory for physiotherapy 175–6
  assessment 208
  energy conservation 201
  lifestyle management 202–3, 206–7
Euthanasia 264
Ex-smokers 23
Exercise
  ability and physiotherapy 156
  acute effects 76
  capacity 14
  dyspnoea 14–15
  intensity and oxygen uptake 68

muscle
   blood flow 69
   oxygen uptake 69
   pH 71
  oxygen
   cost of breathing 74
   uptake response 68–9
   whole-body uptake 68
  performance 6, 66
  prescription for aerobic training 87, **88**, 89–90
  rehabilitation 66
  training 66
  ventilatory reserve 30
  ventilatory response 83
Exercise testing 13
  field tests 31, 32–4, **35**, 37
  laboratory assessment 31–2, 36–7
  maximal incremental 89
  training threshold 36
Exercise tolerance
  assessment 31–7
  COPD 83, 84–5
  endurance test 36–7
  maximal 36
  submaximal 36
Exercise training 14
  assessment 157
  asthma 74
  diary 92
  effective regimen 90
  individual prescription 92
  intensity 89
  maintenance 94
  muscle metabolism 75
  oxygen desaturation 94, **95**
  performance improvement 73
  physiotherapy 157
  programme efficacy assessment 95–6
  specificity 119–20
  strength 76
  studies *78*
  symptom-limited 89
  upper-extremity 123
  see also Aerobic training
Exertion, exhalation 165
Existential distress 263
Expiration, huff 168
Expiratory muscle training 112

Failure, fear of 183
Family
  conflicts 265
  support 262
Fat
  loss in COPD 129
  stores in arm fat area and arm muscle area 142–3
Fat mass 137, 138

assessment 138–9
  change recording 150
  four-site skinfold thickness 141
  redistribution 138
  skinfold thickness 139–40
Fat-free mass 137, 138
  assessment 138–9
  bioelectrical impedance 143
  change recording 150
Fatigue
  COPD 182
  muscle 71
Fear
  attitude changing 172, 173
  expression 261
  failure 183
Feelings, expression 261
Fibrosing alveolitis 22
Fio$_2$ see Fractional concentration of inspired oxygen
    (*Fio$_2$*)
Fitness 82–3
Flow-volume curve, COPD 216
Flutter valve 171
Food
  diary 146, 147
  intake assessment 144–5
Forced expiration technique (FET) 168
Forced expiratory volume in 1 s (FEV$_1$) 4, 6
  COPD 216–17
  decline 217–18
  lung excision effects in emphysema 235
  mortality relationship 13
  Pao$_2$ decline 27–8
  patient categorizing for exercise 91
  prognostic value 217
  smoking cessation 219
  staging system 217
Forced vital capacity 216
Forward lean sitting (FLS) 159–60
  acute exacerbation of condition 162
  side lying 162, **163**
  standing versions 160–1
  supported 160, **163**
Fractional concentration of inspired oxygen (*Fio$_2$*) 229
Fun 174
Functional capacity
  decline in COPD 82
  improvement 13
  peak oxygen consumption (*Vo$_{2peak}$*) 87
Functional impairment 30
Functional Independence Measure *189*
Functional residual capacity (FRC) 29, 100
  COPD 83
  transdiaphragmatic pressure (Pdi) 102

Gas exchange
  alveolar 70

281

assessment 26–8
    submaximal exercise 70
Gastric pressure, balloon catheter assessment 101
Gastrostomy 150
General exercise reconditioning (GER) 110
General practitioner 265–6
Glucose, exercise effects 76, 77
Glycogen phosphorylase 71
Glycolytic enzymes, ventilatory muscles 103, 104
Goals
    COPD 184
    identifying 186, 191, 194
Grabrails 204
Graded exposure 196–7
Grief support 266

Habits
    COPD effects 182–3
    time management 187
Handicap 7
    conceptual framework of breathlessness 246
    reduction 7
    social disadvantage 250
Harris-Benedict equation 148, 149
Head-down position 162
Health care expenditure 15
Health gain 15
Heart rate
    aerobic training 89–90
    exercise performance in COPD 83
Home
    architectural adaptations 210
    rehabilitation 251
    visits 250
Hoover's sign 164
Hospice movement 256, 257–60
    dementia patients 259
    resistance to non-malignant disease patients 258–9
Hospital admission in crisis management 267
Huff 167–8
Humanist approach 190
Humour 174
Hydration 242
Hyperinflation 218
Hyperpnoea
    isocapnoeic 101–2, 106
    muscle endurance tests 101–2
Hypnosis, smoking cessation 221
Hypogammaglobulinaemia 169
Hypoxaemia 26, 28
    COPD 182

Ideal body weight (IBW) 134–5, 136
Impairment 4–5, 7
    conceptual framework of breathlessness 246,
        247–8
    deficiency in the body 247–8

development 5
    rehabilitation 8
Inactivity
    calcium loss from bone 67
    consequences 66
    muscle mass 66–7
    muscle metabolic activity 68
    whole body 67
Inactivity cycle 157
Independence 188
Inhalation, relaxation 165
Inhaler use 248
Inspiratory muscle shortening in COPD 158
Inspiratory muscle training 100
    COPD 108–9
    exercise training effects 110
    functional changes 109–10
    mechanical ventilation weaning 109
    muscle strength 100–1
    MVV 110
    results of programmes 109–11
Inspiratory time (Ti) 102
Insulin, exercise effects 76, 77
Interactive skills 188
Interests
    COPD effects 183
    developing 186
    identifying 191, 194
Intermittent positive pressure ventilation (IPPV) 232,
        233
Internal control maintenance 194–5
Isolated muscle training 118
    practical application 123–4
    specificity 119–20

Joint mobility 174–5

Kielhofner model of human occupation 180, **181**
Kyphoscoliosis 21, 22

Lactate
    blood concentrations in exercise training 74, 75
    blood response in patient categorizing for exercise
        91
    concentration in aerobic exercise 87
    post-exercise response 86
Lactic acid 71
Laughter 174
Legs
    fatigue in COPD 70
    isolated muscle training 123–4
    training 120
    weights 123–4
Leisure activities 188
    maintenance of strength/coordination 206
Leisure facilities, architectural adaptations 210
Leisure restriction 184

Lifestyle management 180–1
  assessment 185
  equipment provision 202–3
  goal identification 191, 194
  interest identification 191, 194
  internal control maintenance 194–5
  outcome evaluation 211
  problem definition 186, *190–1, 192*
  problem-solving *192*, 194–5
  programme implementation 211
  standardized assessments 185, *188–9*
  treatment methods 20–1
  treatment process 185–8, *189–92*
  treatment programme
    implementation 188, 189, 190–1, 194–5
    intervention method 191
    location 191
    planning 186–8
Living pattern, reclusive 158
Living wills 267
  see also Advanced directives
Lobectomy 234
Loss 258
Lower-limb training *see* Legs
Lung
  elasticity 84
  function 216–17
    values 91
  hyperinflation 28, 158
  resection 21
  structure 216
  total capacity 100
  transplantation 21
  volume reduction 235
Lung disease
  advanced and morphine use 269
  breathlessness 6
  clinical features 215–16
  disability development 3–7
  impairment 5
  mortality 13
  pathology 215–16
  social aspects of care 242–3
  social consequences 14
  surgery 233, 233–6
  symptoms 14–15, 271

M-wave 101
Macmillan nurse specialists 257, 262
Mahler baseline and transitional dyspnoea index
    29–30
Maintenance therapy 173, 174
Malnutrition
  clinical appearance 133
  COPD 128–34
  depressed muscle synthesis 130
  energy balance 130–1

food intake 131
  infection susceptibility 130
  malabsorption 131
  nutritional support 148–51
  protein-energy 129
  pulmonary rehabilitation 128
  respiratory muscle effect 130
  reversal in COPD 133–4
  supplemental enteral feeding 150
Manual techniques 175
Marasmus 129
Marital problems 250
Maximal oxygen consumption (Vo_{2max}) 35, 36, 69
  aerobic exercise 95
  aerobic training intensity 90–1
  endurance 72
  exercise intensity 68
  training effects 72
Maximal voluntary ventilation (MVV) 30, 83
  hyperpnoea 101–2
  inspiratory muscle training 110
  ventilatory muscle training 106–7
Maximal work
  intensity in aerobic training 89
  rate 74
Maximum sustained ventilatory capacity (MSVC)
  hyperpnoea 102
  ventilatory muscle training 106
Maximum ventilation (V_{Emax}) 30, 83
Mechanical loading 67
Medical crisis
  management 247–8
  prevention 247–8
Mid-arm circumference (MAC) 141
Mid-arm muscle circumference (MMAC) 141, 142
Mobility resources 248
Money problems 250
Morphine 267, 269
Mortality 13–14
Motivation, rehabilitation programme 39
Motor neurone disease 258
Mouth pressure 101
MRC breathlessness scale 29
Mucolytic drugs 226
Mucus-secreting cells, hypertrophy 166
Multidimensional Functional Assessment
    Questionnaire *189*
Multiple sclerosis 258
Muscle
  aerobic training 84
  blood flow during exercise 69
  contractile apparatus integrity 100
  energy substrate 71
  fatigue 71
    peripheral 84
  fibre types 129
  force of contraction 100

force-frequency relationship 100
force-velocity relationship 100
glycogen depletion 70
length-tension relationship 100
mass and inactivity 66–7
metabolic activity 68
metabolic change, lack in COPD 84–5
metabolism in exercise training 75
oxygen uptake 69
pH in exercise 71
progressive relaxation 196
prolonged isometric contraction 76
Muscle wasting
  COPD 128, 129
  muscle synthesis reduction 129–30
  pink puffer 130
  preferential atrophy of type 2 fibres 129
Muscular impairment in COPD 182
Musculoskeletal problems 175

Nasal intermittent positive pressure ventilation
    (NIPPV) 233
National Institutes of Health workshop 8
Nebulizers 224, 225
  humidification 166
  physiotherapist education role 172
Negative pressure devices 232–3
Neuromuscular disease, inspiratory muscle training 111
Nicotine substitutes 220–1
Nottingham Health Profile 50, *51*
Nursing, rehabilitation 238–9
Nutrient-dense foods 149
Nutrition 128
  adequacy monitoring in COPD 134
  clinical assessment 146–7
  drug history 146–7
  status 144, 145
  support in malnutrition 148–51
Nutritional assessment 134–5, *136*, 137–44
  body composition 137–9
  body weight 134–5, *136*
  intake 144–6
Nutritional supplements 152

Obesity 43
  COPD 147–8
  grading *136*
  pulmonary rehabilitation 128
  target weight 147
Occupational therapy 43, 180–1
  outcome evaluation 211
  process **186**
  treatment methods 20–1
  treatment process 185–8, *189–92*
  treatment programme
    implementation 188, 189, 190–1, 194–5, 211
    planning 186–8

Oesophageal pressure balloon catheter assessment
    101
Older Americans Resources and Services Schedule *189*
Opiates 242
Oral hygiene 242
Out-patient services 20, 92
Oxygen
  ambulatory 230–1
    cylinder provision 94
  concentrator 230
  cost
    diagram 29
    exercise 74
  delivery
    assessment 37
    methods 228–9
  desaturation
    during eating 131
    during training 94, **95**
  dissociation curve **227**
  exercise training 94–5
  fractional concentration of inspired (Fio_2) 229
  partial pressure (Pao_2) 27, 227, 229
  portable 230–1
  saturation 28
    pursed-lips breathing 165
  supplementary delivery 228–9
  supply methods 228–9
  symptomatic treatment 229
  systems and physiotherapist education role 172
  tissue delivery 227–8
  transtracheal delivery 229
  uptake response to exercise 69
Oxygen consumption (Vo_2) 35
  arm activity 119
  indirect measures in aerobic training 87
  patient categorizing for exercise 91
  see also Maximal oxygen consumption (Vo_{2max}); Peak
    oxygen consumption (Vo_{2peak})
Oxygen consumption (Vo_2)/heart rate slope 83
Oxygen therapy 9, 12, 226–31
  air travel 232
  flow rate 230
  long-term (LTOT) 229–30, 247
Oxygen-dependent patients 23

$Paco_2$ *see* Carbon dioxide arterial partial pressure
    ($Paco_2$)
Pain
  management strategies 270
  reduction 174–5
  total 260–1
Palliation 256
Palliative care
  bereavement support 266
  crisis management 267
  expression of feelings 261

family conflicts 265
family support 262
hospital-based 259
multidisciplinary teamwork 262
patient concerns 261
planning terminal care 263–5
primary care team 265–6
specific symptoms 267–8
symptom control 260–1
terminal stage acceptance 264
see also Terminal care
Pao_2 *see* Oxygen, partial pressure (Pao_2)
Patient
   autonomy 259
   characteristics 40
   exclusion 23
   selection 20–3
Patient assessment 23, *24*, 25–43
   data requirements *26*
   exercise tolerance 31–7
   gas exchange 26–8
   individual treatment 42–3
   likely to graduate from rehabilitation programme
      39–42
   objectives 23, 25
   oxygen delivery 37
   physiological data 25–31
   respiratory muscle strength 37
   signs/symptoms 25–31
Patient-provider relationship 39
Peak flow measurement in asthma 216
Peak oxygen consumption (Vo_{2peak}) 35, 36, 69, 74
   aerobic training 87
   exercise intensity 68
Performance skills 182–3
Phosphofructokinase 71
Phrenic nerve stimulation, bilateral simultaneous
    transcutaneous 101
Physical performance decline 20
Physician role in rehabilitation programmes 214–15
Physiotherapy 42–3, 156
   accessory equipment 175–6
   attitude changing 172–4
   education 171–4
   group programmes 162
   joint mobility 174–5
   pain reduction 174–5
   positioning 158–62, **163**
   secretion clearance 165–71
   techniques 157–62, **163**, 164–71
Pink puffer 229
   muscle wasting 130
Platypnoea 218
Pleural surface pressure change 101
Pneumonectomy 234
Polio 232
Polycythaemia 218

Positioning 158–62, **163**
   gravity-assisted 169
   head-down 162
   minimizing breathlessness 241
Positive expiratory pressure (PEEP) 170–1
Postural drainage 169
Prealbumin 138
Prednisolone 225
Primary care team role 265–6
Problem solving, patient discharge from hospital 243
Progesterone 226
Progressive muscular relaxation 196
Project 2000 239
Protein
   dietary intake 148–9
   skeletal 138
   stores in arm fat area and arm muscle area 142–3
   visceral 138, 144
Protein-energy malnutrition 129
Psychological distress 271
Psychologist 43
Pulmonary fibrosis development 3
Pulmonary hypertension 182
Pulmonary rehabilitation programmes *see*
    Rehabilitation

Quadriplegia, inspiratory muscle training 111
Quality of life 13, 14–15
   assessment 37–8, 50
   asthma 58
   behaviour pattern 59
   biological condition improvement 59–60
   change 57–9
   construct classification 57
   content-valid instruments 56
   deficits 50
   disease-specific instruments 50, 52–4, **55**, 56–7
   domain classification 57
   emotional problems 57, 58
   estimates 9
   generic scale 57, 59
   health-related 38
   improving 59–60
   maintenance of benefit 15–16
   multicomponent concept 59
   outcome 60
   patient-generated constructs 57
   physical problems 57, 585
   psychological constructs **58**
   questionnaires 38, 50
   researcher-generated domains 56–7
   treatment effects 58
   upper-extremity training 122

Radiography 216
Rand Functional Limitations Battery *189*
Reassurance 172–3

Referral 20–1
Rehabilitation 2–3, 240
  assessment 11, 23, *24*, 25–43
    objectives 23, 25
  at home 246–51
  components 10–12
  contributors to programme 11
  coordination 11
  definitions 8–9
  disability reduction 4
  disease education 214–15
  effectiveness 13–15
  exercise tests 13
  group programmes 162
  individual treatment 42–3
  intervention 60
  maintenance of benefit 15–16
  nursing 238–9
  nutritional assessment 134–5, *136*, 137–44
  out-patient 92
  outcome measures 11, 12–13
  physiological functioning 59
  physiotherapy role 156–7
  process 9–10
  programme 11–12
    audit 44
    compliance 39–42
    cost-benefit analysis 44
    goals 41
    management nutrition 144–51
    motivation 39
    patients likely to graduate 39–42
    structure 22
    tailoring 41
  psychological functioning 59
  quality of life 13
  respiratory nurse 240
  selection procedure 11–12
  service evaluation 44
  setting 10–11
  structure 10–12
  target 7
  upper-extremity training 120–3
  variety of training 86
Rehousing 204
Relaxation
  anxiety management 196
  inhalation 165
  progressive muscular 196
  strategies 248
Religious aspects 263
Residual volume (RV) 100
Resistive loading, muscle endurance 102
Respiratory disease, air travel 231–2
Respiratory failure
  definition 227
  management 228

Respiratory medicine 9, 239
Respiratory muscle
  chronic weakness 233
  COPD 70, 108–9
  diseases associated with weakness *105*
  endurance 101–3, 108
  fibre types 103–5
  function coordination 112
  histochemical composition 103–5
  length 100
  malnutrition 130
  maximal static contractions 103, **104**
  respiratory load response 108
  strength evaluation 37, 100–1
  training 100
    hyperpnoeic 106
    methods 106–7
    rationale 105–6
    response 107–8
Respiratory nurse 238
  breathless patient in hospital 241–2
  breathlessness management 240–1
  communication 242
  patient discharge from hospital 242–6
  practice 240–1
  professional issues 246
  rehabilitation 240
    at home 246–51
  role 239–40, 251
  team work 240
  therapeutic plan 242
Respiratory stimulants 242
Respite care 251
  hospices 258
Responsibilities, adaptations 184
Resting energy expenditure (REE) 132–3, 148
Retinol-binding protein 138
Ribcage paradox 218
Roles
  assessment 188
  COPD effects 182–3
  current/future 204
Rollator frames 176

St George's Respiratory Questionnaire 38, 50, *52*, 53–4, 56, 60
  subscales 56–7
Salbutamol *222*, 223
Scoliosis 21, 233
  paralytic 232
Secretion clearance 156, 165–71
  active cycle of breathing techniques (ACBT) 167–8
  autogenic drainage 168–9
  chest clapping 169–70
  chest compression with shaking and/or vibration 170
  humidification 166–7

positive expiratory pressure (PEEP) 170–1
postural drainage 169
Self talk 197
Self-care 188
    maintenance of strength/coordination 206
Self-compression 170
Self-esteem 66, 183, 184
    loss 201
    low 209
Self-help group 15, 16, 173, 174, 250
    stop smoking 23
Self-medication 244
Self-neglect 266
Self-reporting 42
Self-worth 183
Sex therapy 43
Sexual activity 204
    medications effects 206
    physical functioning 205
    psychological state 206
Shopping trolley 160–1
Short Form-36 50, *51*
Shoulder girdle
    fixing 158–9, 159–60
    relaxation 160
    support posture 218
Shuttle walking
    aerobic training 87
    test 33, **35**, 59
Sickness Impact Profile 50, *51*
Sitting, forward lean position 159–60
Skeletal protein 138
Skinfold anthropometry 138, 139–43
    reproducibility 140
    serial change of index 143
Skinfold thickness
    four-site 141
    measurement sites **140**
    triceps and mid-arm muscle circumference 141–2
Sleep apnoea 182
Slow-twitch fibres 103
Smoking 2
    anaesthesia risk 234
    cessation 219–21
        nicotine substitutes 220–1
    COPD 218
    guilt 263
    lung impairment 5
    patient selection 22
    patients in rehabilitation programmes 215
    surgery risk 234
Social contact, limited 209–10
Social function 15
Social Security benefits 209
Social workers 265, 266
Somatic factors, patient compliance 40
Speech impairment 210

Spiritual distress 263
Spirometry 21, 216
Sputum production 165
Standardized assessments in lifestyle management
    185, *188–9*
Steam inhalation 166, **167**
Step test 34
    constant 37
Steroids
    inhaled 221
    obesity 147
Strength training 76, 121–3
Stress
    inoculation training 197
    psychosocial 258
Stroke volume, aerobic exercise 84
Suicide
    assisted 264
    risk 266
Support groups 173, 174, 234
Surgery 233–6
    lung volume reduction 235
Sustainable inspiratory pressure (SIP) 102–3
Symptom control 267–71

Task magnitude 30
Teamwork, multidisciplinary 262
Telemetry, short-range 25, **26**
Terbutaline *222*, 223
Terminal care 256–7
    planning 263–5
    see also Palliative care
Terminal stage acceptance 264
Tetraplegia, inspiratory muscle training 111
Theophyllines *222*, 223
Therapeutic plan 242
Thoracic expansion 167, 168
Thoracic spine disorders 21
Thoracic surgery 234
    emphysema 234–5
    lung volume reduction 235
Thought processes, awareness 197
Threshold loading 102–3
Ti/Ttot ratio 102
Tidal volume
    controlled breathing 162
    pursed-lips breathing 165
Time management 187
    delegation 201
    education 198–9
    objectives 199
    planning 199–200
    self-objectives 200–1
    steps 199–201
Time saving, home 249
Total body water (TBW) 137
    bioelectrical impedance 143, 144

Total lung capacity (TLC) 100
Total pain concept 260–1
Training 66
    specificity 119–20
Transdiaphragmatic pressure (Pdi) 101, 102
Transfer factor for lung carbon monoxide (TLCO) 6
Transferrin 138
    visceral protein status 144
Treadmill test 32, 36
Treatment process 185–8
Triceps skinfold (TSF) thickness 141–2
Triglycerides 76, 77
Tuberculosis 3
    family visitor 239
Tumour necrosis factor 133

UK Central Council 239
UK National Council for Hospices and Palliative Care
        Services 257
Underweight 43
Upper-extremity training 118–20
    breathlessness 118–19
    exercise 123
    rehabilitation 120–3
    specificity 119–20
    strength training 121–3
    supported vs unsupported arm training 121
    weight training 122–3, 123–4
    see also Arm training

Values, COPD effects 183
V_{Emax} see Maximum ventilation (V_{Emax})
Ventilatory disease, non-obstructive 111
Ventilatory drive 28

Ventilatory load in arm activity 119
Ventilatory mechanics 70
Ventilatory support 9
    non-invasive 232–3
Visceral protein 138
    status 144
Visual analogue scale (VAS) 30
    symptom-limited exercise training 89
Vo_{2max} see Maximal oxygen consumption (Vo_{2max})
Vo_{2peak} see Peak oxygen consumption (Vo_{2peak})
Vo_2 see Oxygen consumption (Vo_2)
Volition 183–4

Walking 86
    ability tests 32–3, 35
    distance in upper-extremity training 122
    endurance 35
    frames 176
    metabolic rate 68
    programme **93**, 94
    stick 160, 176
    test performance 14
Water see Total body water (TBW)
Weight loss 218
    treatment 131–2
Weight training
    chronic airflow limitation 122–3
    isolated muscle training 123–4
Work activity 188
    energy conservation of methods 201–2
    maintenance of strength/coordination 206
Work facility adaptations 210
Work rate 74
Working conditions, anger 263